Lessons from

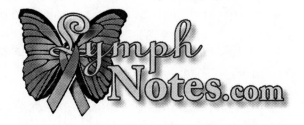

Advanced praise for *Living Well With Lymphedema*:

"This book is very well organized and thought out, providing enough detail, explanation, and practical insight to enable someone with lymphedema to live safely and well. I definitely recommend it to anyone with, or at risk for, lymphedema."
John Giusto, MD

"After two years of treatment with an outstanding therapist, I know a lot about my condition and my role in managing it. But I learned something new on every page of this book. It will be a wonderful reference for me as a periodic check of my self-management."
Dixie Lee Spiegel, PhD

"This book is upbeat and positive while dealing with a condition that can be overwhelming."
Deborah G. Kelly, PT, MSEd, CLT-LANA, Associate Professor at the University of Kentucky and author of a textbook for lymphedema therapists

"The most comprehensive lymphedema book on the market. Wonderful for patients and those at risk. So many sources tell lymphedema patients what they can't do. This book encourages us in what we can do! I absolutely loved the chapter on emotional challenges. Finally I feel that someone understands and then provides me with appropriate coping suggestions and alternatives. Thanks."
Tracy Novak, post mastectomy lymphedema patient and founder of the West Virginia Support Network

"This book is a resource I can enthusiastically recommend to my patients. The content is up-to-date, comprehensive, and well illustrated. It reinforces what I teach my patients and answers the questions they forget to ask."
Doris Laing, CLT-LANA

"What a gift these authors have given to anyone affected with lymphedema! One of the most thorough and informative books I have ever read."
Debbie Robinson, concerned family member

Living Well With
Lymphedema

by
Ann Ehrlich
Alma Vinjé-Harrewijn, PT, CLT
Elizabeth McMahon, PhD

Lymph Notes
San Francisco

Living Well With Lymphedema
© 2005 by Lymph Notes

Lymph Notes
2929 Webster Street
San Francisco, CA 94123 USA
www.LymphNotes.com   sales@lymphnotes.com

Notice of Rights

Notice of Liability

Trademarks

ISBN 0-9764806-1-1
Library of Congress Control Number: 2005921672
Publishing history—first edition, printing 1.02

Cover pastel by Patty Rice, www.pattyrice.com

Preface

The Epidemic No One Talks About

Now that cancer has become a chronic condition, we face a stealth epidemic of lymphedema among cancer survivors. Many physicians don't recognize lymphedema and some deny that it happens—but there it is in all of its swollen glory. That is the gloomy side of the picture.

The bright side of this picture is that this is changing! Physicians and other healthcare providers are becoming more aware of lymphedema and promising research on lymphedema prevention and treatment is underway. Most importantly there is a growing—but still not large enough—pool of specialized therapists who treat lymphedema and improve the quality of life for their patients.

Another change for the better is that patients are taking a more active role in the management of their own healthcare. These patients ask questions and search for answers. They want to know! Many also support each other by swapping tips on what works, or doesn't work, or just by listening through the tough times that come from living with a chronic condition.

Our goal is to provide practical information in a format that is easy-to-understand for people with lymphedema, friends and family, and healthcare professionals. We hope that we will be able to help you live well with lymphedema.

Acknowledgements

Many of those who are living with lymphedema have shared their thoughts on the Lymph Notes web site. Their insights and ability to live well with lymphedema are an inspiration to us all. To each we say, *"Thank you for helping each other, the authors, and ultimately the readers of this book."*

I want to thank my family for their love, help, and support as together we have learned how to live well with lymphedema. I also want to thank the lymphedema therapists who have skillfully and gently treated me over the years. They continue to play a key role in my well-being and quality of life.
—Ann

I gained a wealth of experience from the many patients I have treated over the years. More importantly, I have come to respect their valor in learning to live with lymphedema. Being part of a team and working together to create this book has been an exciting new experience for me. Thank you for inviting me to participate in this project. Last, but not least, I want to thank Jan for his love and support.
—Alma

I want to acknowledge my wonderful co-authors, without whom this book would not exist, and my patients whose courage in coping with physical and emotional challenges fills me with respect. Thanks also to my extended family who are models for facing and coping with life's difficulties. And thank you, from my heart, to my husband for his love and help.
—Elizabeth

The authors thank the many people who have worked with us to make this book a reality beginning with Debbie and Cliff who read the very first rough drafts and asked the *"lymph-a-what?"* questions. We are grateful to our reviewers for their insights, suggestions, and attention to detail. Each of them played an important role in shaping this book:

- **John Giusto, MD**, specialist in physical medicine and rehabilitation, Plum Spring Clinic.

- **Melissa A. Green, MPH**, lymphedema patient, public health educator, and coordinator of the Duke University Health Inequalities Program.

- **Deborah G. Kelly, MSEd, CLT-LANA**, Associate Professor at University of Kentucky and author of **A Primer on Lymphedema**.

- **Doris Laing, CLT-LANA**, a lymphedema therapist with extensive experience and infinite patience in answering questions.

- **Nancy Mize, PhD**, pharmacogenomics and proteomics specialist at Pacific BioDevelopment.

- **Tracy Novak**, lymphedema patient, activist, and founder of the West Virginia Lymphedema Network.

- **Dixie Lee Spiegel, PhD**, Professor of Literacy Studies at UNC School of Education and a lymphedema patient.

The authors wish to thank Barbara Abercrombie for allowing them to excerpt parts of her experience with lymphedema as it was told in her book **Writing Out the Storm: Reading and Writing Your Way Through Serious Illness or Injury** (published by St. Martin's Press, 2002) as Barbara's Story.

The authors wish to thank the individuals and companies that helped make this a better book by providing illustrations:

- **Figures 1-1, 3-3, 3-6, 6-1, 9-1, 10-43, 11-4,** and **11-6** are photo illustrations based on photos by Alma Vinjé-Harrewijn.

- **Figure 2-1,** pitting edema photos courtesy of H.P.M. Verdonk. Reprinted with permission from **Oedeem en Oedeemtherapie** by H.P.M. Verdonk, et al. Bohn Stafleu and Van Loghum (www.bsl.nl) 2000, p. 48.

- **Figure 2-2** is courtesy of Lymflo Therapies, Chapel Hill, NC.

- **Figure 3-1** is a photo illustration based on a photo by J. J. Vinjé.

- **Figure 3-2** bandaging photo courtesy of BSN-Jobst, Inc. www.jobst-usa.com.

- **Figure 3-4** compression aid photo courtesy of Peninsula Medical, Inc. www.lymphedema.com.

- **Figure 3-5** sequential pneumatic pump photo courtesy of Lympha Press® Compression Therapy Systems, www.lympha-press.com.

- **Figures 11-1, 11-2, 11-3,** and **11-5,** bandaging supplies photos courtesy of BSN-Jobst, Inc. www.jobst-usa.com.

- **Figure 11-7** electric bandage winder photo courtesy of Bandages Plus, www.bandagesplus.com.

- **Figures 10-1** and **IV-1 to IV-11** are based on artwork licensed from Giunti International, www.giunti.it.

- **Figures 10-2 to 10-39** and **12-1 to 12-7** are photo illustrations based on photos by Chuck Ehrlich.

- **Figures 10-40 to 10-42** are photo illustrations based on a photo by Philip Greenspun.

- **Cover art** is a pastel by Patty Rice, www.pattyrice.com.

Table of Contents

Contents in Brief

Contents in Detail

How to Use This Book

Your need to know about lymphedema depends on your situation. You may be interested in our suggested reading paths for:

- Recently diagnosed with lymphedema, see page 2.

- People at risk of developing lymphedema, see page 3.

- Veterans of living with lymphedema, see page 4.

- Health professionals and caregivers, see page 5.

- Family and friends, see page 6.

Alternatively you can start by using the table of contents or index to locate topics of interest to you or just start reading.

We also suggest checking the Lymph Notes web site (www.lymphnotes.com) for additional information and our online lymphedema support group.

If You are Recently Diagnosed with Lymphedema

☐ **Study the "Protect Yourself"** guidelines on page 7. These precautions are important to your well being!

☐ **Read Section II—Understanding Lymphedema.** Here you will find the answers to many of your current questions.

☐ **Study Section IV—Understanding the Lymphatic System.** Here you will learn about this very important body system and the ways in which lymphedema treatment works with the unique flow of lymph.

☐ **Read Section III—Self-Management of Lymphedema.** After you have started treatment, you will play an important role in the successful treatment of your lymphedema. This section should reinforce the self-management information provided by your therapist.

If You are at Risk of Developing Lymphedema

☐ **Study the "Protect Yourself"** guidelines on page 7. It is important that you follow these precautions because they may prevent you from developing lymphedema.

☐ **Read Chapter 1—What is Lymphedema** to learn why you are at risk for secondary lymphedema and why you will remain at risk.

☐ **Read Chapter 2—How Lymphedema is diagnosed.** Pay close attention to the *"Early Warning Signs of Lymphedema."* Should any of these signs develop, seek a diagnosis and treatment immediately. Chapter 4 explains where to find treatment.

☐ **Read Chapter 6—Complications of Lymphedema.** Infections are a major lymphedema complication that can suddenly become medical emergencies. A complication may be the first sign that you have developed lymphedema and you will want to know what to do if this happens.

☐ **Read Section IV—Understanding the Lymphatic System.** Learn more about how this body system works and why you are at risk for developing lymphedema.

☐ **Save this book and review it periodically!** Should you develop lymphedema, follow the suggestions for the "Recently Diagnosed."

If You are a Long-Time Veteran of Lymphedema

☐ **Study the "Protect Yourself"** guidelines on page 7. It is still important that you follow these precautions.

☐ **Read Section III—Self-Management of Lymphedema.** This will help you review your self-management program. If you still have questions, ask your therapist to review these steps with you again.

☐ **Read Section II—Understanding Lymphedema.** Learn about the current treatment recommendations and standards for lymphedema therapists, plus practical suggestions on how to appeal if your health insurance company denies treatment.

☐ **Study Section IV—Understanding the Lymphatic System** to learn how the treatment of lymphedema works with the unique structure of the lymphatic system.

If You are a Caregiver or Healthcare Professional

☐ **Study the "Protect Yourself"** guidelines on page 7. Always follow these guidelines when working with someone who has lymphedema or is at risk of developing it.

☐ **Read Section II—Understanding Lymphedema** to gain insights into lymphedema, how it is diagnosed, frequent complications, current treatment methods, and training standards for lymphedema therapists.

☐ **If you are a caregiver, Section III—Self-Management of Lymphedema** is essential reading. You may be responsible for carrying out the self-management program. If you have questions about this care, ask the client's therapist for specific details.

☐ **Read Section IV—Understanding the Lymphatic System** to learn more about how the functioning of the lymphatic system influences the treatment of lymphedema.

If You are a Concerned Family Member or Friend

☐ **Study the "Protect Yourself"** guidelines on page 7. These guidelines must be followed whenever medical care is provided for someone with lymphedema, or someone who is at risk for developing lymphedema.

☐ **Read Section II—Understanding Lymphedema** to gain insights into lymphedema, how it is diagnosed, frequent complications, current treatment methods and training standards for lymphedema therapists.

☐ **Read Section III—Self-Management of Lymphedema.** There are many ways in which you can help with this phase of treatment. It may be by assisting with self-massage or self-bandaging. Also providing support and motivation in keeping up with the exercise program is very important. If you have questions about this care, ask the patient's therapist for specific details.

☐ **Read Section IV—Understanding the Lymphatic System** to learn more about how the functioning of the lymphatic system influences the treatment of lymphedema.

Protect Yourself !

If you have lymphedema, or are at risk of developing lymph-edema, follow these guidelines to protect yourself:

☐ **Avoid having a blood pressure reading on the affected limb.** The blood pressure cuff can alter or damage lymphatic function within the area.

☐ **Avoid any injection, blood draw, finger prick, or IV placement in the affected limb.** Any break in the skin can lead to an infection.

☐ **Avoid having acupuncture needles placed in the affected limb.** Although these are very fine needles, they still break the skin.

☐ **Protect the affected area to prevent injuries, sunburn, or insect bites that can damage the skin.** When outside wear protective clothing, sunscreen, and insect repellent.

☐ **Maintain a normal weight.** Being even slightly over-weight increases your risk of developing secondary lymphedema.

☐ **Wear a compression garment when flying.** Changes in cabin pressure can increase the swelling of lymphedema. Also, these pressure changes may trigger the initial onset of lymphedema.

Understanding Lymphedema

Recommended Reading

Section IV—Understanding the Lymphatic System will help you understand the causes of lymphedema and the ways in which lymphedema is treated. You will also want to refer to this section as questions arise.

Pam's Story, Part I

To celebrate the completion of her breast cancer treatments, Pam flew to Hawaii for a relaxing two week vacation. During the return flight, the arm next to her treated area began to ache and swell.

The swelling did not go away after she got home, and soon Pam was back in her oncologist's office. Dr. Metzger's diagnosis was lymphedema and she immediately referred Pam for treatment.

While waiting for her first visit at the *"Here for You"* lymphedema treatment center, Pam was surprised to find herself seated next to a teenage girl who was engrossed in listening to her iPod®. Pam noticed a thick stocking peeking out from under one leg of her jeans. A well-dressed businessman was seated across the room, to Pam's surprise, a therapist came out and escorted him in for treatment.

After she finished her new-patient paperwork, Pam wondered what the three of them could possibly have in common. Soon, a pleasant therapist called Pam's name and introduced herself as Tracy. Thus began Pam's introduction into the world of lymphedema. Soon she would learn that lymphedema was the bond she shared with the teen, the businessman, and millions of others.

continued on page 118

Chapter 1

What is Lymphedema?

Lymphedema Defined

Lymphedema, or *lymphoedema*, is abnormal swelling that occurs when the lymphatic system fails to develop properly or has been damaged. Lymphedema is a chronic and degenerative condition. Although lymphedema cannot currently be cured, it can be managed by ongoing treatment.

Without effective treatment, the lymphatic swelling increases and causes the tissues to harden. This swollen skin, which has lost its flexibility, hangs in folds and frequently develops cracks or sores that increase the risk of infection. Uncontrolled lymphedema may result in life threatening infections, disfigurement, the loss of mobility, and total disability.

With early and ongoing treatment, the progression of the disease can be slowed significantly and deterioration may be prevented. The sooner treatment begins, the better the chances of a successful outcome.

Different Kinds of Swelling

Swelling, or *edema*, is the body's normal response to an injury such as a sprain. This swelling is caused by protein-poor tissue fluid flowing into the area as part of the healing process. As healing progresses, the excess fluid leaves the area and the swelling goes down. The swelling of lymphedema does not work in this manner.

The swelling of lymphedema is caused by lymph that is unable to drain from the tissues normally. This protein-rich fluid creates an ideal breeding ground for bacteria. If bacteria enter through a break in the skin, they multiply rapidly in the lymph and can quickly cause a life-threatening infection. How lymph becomes protein-rich is explained in "Understanding the Lymphatic System" (Section IV). Infections due to bacteria entering the tissues are discussed in Chapter 6.

The Types of Lymphedema

The types of lymphedema discussed in this book are **primary lymphedema** and **secondary lymphedema**. Primary lymphedema is a hereditary disorder and secondary lymphedema develops as a result of damage to the lymphatic system. Treatment for these two forms of lymphedema is the same, even though they have different causes.

Primary Lymphedema

Primary lymphedema is an inherited disorder that affects somewhere between one in every 6,000 to one in every 300 people at birth.[1,2]

Often, there is a family history of several generations of family members, usually female, having a "fat leg." More frequently, the family history is incomplete because earlier cases of lymphedema were not diagnosed.

Primary lymphedema is caused by malformation of the lymphatic vessels and the characteristic swelling typically begins at the foot and progresses upward toward the trunk.[3] This swelling can be seen in Figure 1-1. Primary lymphedema, which can develop at any age, is further classified by the age at which it appears.[4]

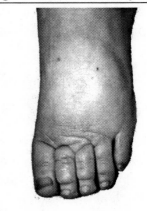

Figure 1-1: Swelling of the toes and foot due to primary lymphedema

---

How common is Lymphedema?

US Department of Health and Human Services estimates:

- Primary lymphedema occurs in between 1/6,000 and 1/300 live births. This implies 50,000 to 1,000,000 gene carriers in the US.

- Secondary lymphedema affects 3-5 million people in the US.

This secondary lymphedema estimate is consistent with the Centers for Disease Control and Prevention estimate of 10 million cancer survivors in the US and a 20-40% incidence of lymphedema in cancer survivors, plus some number of people with secondary lymphedema due to other causes.

The World Health Organization estimates that 170 million people have secondary lymphedema worldwide. This estimate includes about 120 million cases of lymphatic filariasis, implying about 50 million people have secondary lymphedema from other causes.

Congenital Lymphedema

Congenital lymphedema, also known as *Milroy's syndrome,* is present at birth or develops within the first two years of life.[5] Sometimes swelling of the toes can be identified on a prenatal sonogram. This swelling requires further diagnostic investigation soon after birth because it could be a symptom of other conditions such as Turner syndrome.[6] *Turner syndrome,* which affects only females, is a hereditary condition caused by a missing or defective chromosome.

Lymphedema Praecox

Lymphedema praecox, also known as *Meige Disease,* is primary lymphedema that appears between puberty and the age of 35. Approximately 75 percent of all primary lymphedema cases develop during this age span with the

---

Stories of Lymph Notes Members

- Lymphedema runs in my family. My grandmother has a very severe case. One of my aunts has it, and so do a few others who are overweight.

- I am, at least, a third generation in my family suffering from this condition. I've had primary lymphedema since I was 13 and now I am 25 years old.

- I was diagnosed with primary lymphedema in both legs during my freshman year of college; however, I successfully played volleyball for 4 years of college and am now attending graduate school.

---

majority occuring during adolescence. This condition occurs in four times as many females as males and it usually affects only one leg.[7]

Lymphedema Tarda

Lymphedema tarda develops after the age of 35 with swelling in one or both legs.[8] It affects both males and females; however, it too occurs most frequently in females. The onset of lymphedema tarda is usually sudden and of unknown cause. In some cases there may be a minor incident, such as an insect bite, followed by the swelling of the affected limb. Although the insect bite heals, the swelling does not go away.

Secondary Lymphedema

Secondary lymphedema is an acquired disorder caused by damage to the lymphatic system, with cancer treatment being the largest single cause of secondary lymphedema in developed countries. (Lymphatic filariasis, a tropical disease caused by a parasite, is a different condition and is not covered in this book.)

Secondary lymphedema develops adjacent to the lymphatic structures that have been removed or damaged. It can develop in all parts of the body; however, the arms and legs are the most commonly affected areas.

Risk Factors for Secondary Lymphedema

A person is at risk of developing secondary lymphedema when any of the following potential causes are part of his or her medical history:

- Cancer treatments that disrupt the flow of lymph in the treated area due to lymph node removal (dissection), lymph node biopsy, mastectomy or other surgery, radiation therapy, and/or chemotherapy.

- Burns that damage or destroy lymphatic capillaries located in, and just under, the skin (for example, Sam's story on page 16).

- Scars from any cause that block the normal flow of lymph.

- Excess weight that places additional stress on the lymphatic system (see Chapter 7).

- Circulatory conditions that cause swelling in the feet and legs placing added stress on the lymphatic system (see Chapter 7).

- Fractures, joint dislocations, or other injuries that damage lymphatic tissues or place pressure on lymph vessels.

- Paralysis, multiple sclerosis, inactivity, or other conditions that reduce muscle movement, decrease the normal muscle and joint pump action that aids the flow of lymph (see Section IV—Understanding the Lymphatic System).

Sam's Story

Sam is a workplace safety consultant helping manufacturing companies create safer workplaces for their employees. Having just returned from a client meeting, Sam was dressed for that role as he waited for his lymphedema treatment at *"Here for You."*

Consulting was a new career for Sam, who had previously been a fireman. He used to joke that some little boys dream of becoming firemen and claimed that he never outgrew that dream. Instead he made it come true. All of that changed two years ago when he was pinned to the floor by a burning timber while fighting a massive factory blaze.

Sam's leg was severely burned and badly injured. He survived the burns, overcame the injuries, and regained most of his mobility. He couldn't return to fighting fires but he liked his new career as a consultant. Then "it happened." After a strenuous session of shooting hoops with his buddies, Sam noticed that his injured leg was sore and swollen. He kept trying to ignore it, but the swelling didn't go away.

Sam's doctor, who had treated him since the accident, looked at the swelling and knew what it was. Sam had developed secondary lymphedema due to the scars from his burns and injuries. Now Sam is learning how to manage, and live with, this chronic condition.

Delayed Onset of Secondary Lymphedema

The lymphatic system works to maintain a delicate balance between the flow of fluids into and out of the tissues. As long as this normal balance is maintained, lymphedema-related swelling does not develop. The time between the damage to the lymphatic system and the appearance of the lymphedema symptoms is known as the *latency phase.*[9]

Some therapists describe this situation as being like a bathtub with a clogged drain and a dripping faucet. All is well until the tub becomes full. Then the next drop of water causes the tub to begin overflowing.[10] It is at this point that the swelling of lymphedema appears. For this reason, the onset of lymphedema does not always occur immediately after the causative event. Instead, it can develop months or even years later.

Can Secondary Lymphedema Be Prevented?

Approximately 30 percent of those who are at risk for developing secondary lymphedema will actually go on to develop this condition. However, there are no accurate predictors as to who will or will not develop the condition. Cases of lymphedema developing as long as 30 years after the event that caused the risk have been documented. For this reason, everyone with a lymphedema risk factor is considered to be at risk throughout their lives.

There are many recommended steps thought to prevent the onset of secondary lymphedema. Some of these measures, such as those listed in the chart "Protect Yourself" on page 7, are evidence based. The effectiveness of other suggested precautions has not been as well-documented. However, they are worth paying attention to if there is a reasonable chance that they will prevent the onset of lymphedema. The National Lymphedema Network (www.lymphnet.org) is an excellent resource for more precautions that can be taken in the hope of preventing the onset of secondary lymphedema.

Determining which preventive steps to follow is a personal decision and you may change your mind over time. However, it is important to remember that once you are at risk for developing lymphedema, you always remain at risk.

The tips for those who are at risk for developing lymphedema also contribute to a healthy lifestyle. If you choose to follow this advice, you will be making choices that benefit your health and well-being, even if you never develop lymphedema.

Barbara's Story, Part I—Discovery

An early-June afternoon, two months before my wedding to R., and I'm driving around doing errands. Life is good, and I'm grateful. The wedding invitations are at the printer. I've hired a caterer and arranged for the music. Tonight I'm going out to dinner with the Bosom Buddies (my breast cancer support group).

Last weekend we arranged to have my wedding ring made. As I think about this, happy about the ring, I glance at my left hand on the steering wheel and notice it's puffy. Ominously puffy. It looks like a pincushion without the pins. All the bones and veins in my left hand have suddenly disappeared.

I know instantly what's happened. I think it's lymphedema -- a disfiguring swelling that comes from lymph fluid not being able to drain properly. I've read long lists of warnings for breast cancer patients to avoid the possibility of it suddenly appearing. You can get it immediately after surgery or radiation, or even years later. To avoid it, you're not to carry anything heavy on the side you had surgery, nor have blood pressure taken on that side, no IVs, no tight rings, always wear gloves gardening, beware of high altitudes and sun, take care of burns and scratches that could become infected. In other words, your arm should be placed in bubble wrap for the rest of your life.

continued on page 26

Chapter 2

The Diagnosis of Lymphedema

Do I Have Lymphedema?

If you have any of the warning signs of lymphedema listed below, consult your healthcare professional immediately to have the condition diagnosed.

Warning Signs of the Onset of Lymphedema

☐ An infection within the "at risk" area

☐ Swelling, no matter how slight

☐ Pitting edema as shown in Figure 2-1 (page 22)

☐ An unexplained sensation of "pins and needles"

☐ A feeling of heaviness in the arm or leg

☐ A sensation of tightness in the skin

☐ Changes such as a bracelet or ring that is too tight

☐ One shoe that is suddenly too small or a sleeve that is too tight

☐ Aching in the shoulder or hip joint

☐ Decreased mobility of a joint

At this visit, be sure to mention to your physician that you are at risk for lymphedema.

Who Diagnoses Lymphedema?

People often ask, *"Which medical specialist should I see to diagnose this condition?"* Often the diagnosis is made by the primary care provider, oncologist, or pediatrician who is overseeing the patient's care. Complex cases may be referred to a lymphologist for confirmation or treatment. A *lymphologist* is a physician with specialized training in the diagnosis and treatment of the disorders of the lymphatic system. There are very few lymphologists in the United States; consequently a person may be referred to a vascular surgeon or a specialist in a related field.

After a diagnosis of lymphedema has been made, the patient is usually referred to a qualified lymphedema therapist for an evaluation and ongoing treatment. While being treated by a lymphedema therapist, the patient's care remains under the supervision of the referring physician.

How is Lymphedema Diagnosed?

Approximately 90 percent of all lymphedema cases are diagnosed on the basis of the medical history and current symptoms, which may include complications of lymphedema. The remaining 10 percent of cases require more complex diagnostic measures.

When lymphedema is present in conjunction with another disorder, such as a heart condition, it is essential that the more serious condition be diagnosed and treated first.

The Family History

Because primary lymphedema is a hereditary disorder, the family history is an important diagnostic factor when identifying this condition. Even without a family history that includes documented cases, if swelling of the legs

> *Warning:* There are non-physician practitioners who use the title of *"Certified Lymphologist"* to describe their alternative medicine treatment of the lymphatic system. These practitioners are not qualified to diagnose lymphedema or to refer patients for lymphedema treatment.

due to an unknown cause is present, primary lymphedema cannot be completely ruled out.

The Medical History

Secondary lymphedema is considered when the patient's medical history includes any of the risk factors described in Chapter 1. Because of the delayed onset of secondary lymphedema, these risk factors are not necessarily of recent origin.

The Patient Interview

In preparation for this diagnostic visit, you should prepare a list of any lymphedema warning signs, symptoms, and other recent changes you've noticed. This list should also note the factors that place you at risk of developing secondary lymphedema. (For tips on how to prepare this list, see Chapter 15.) This advance preparation is helpful to you and to your physician.

The Physical Examination

- **Swelling** is the most obvious sign of lymphedema; however, as already noted, not all swelling is due to lymphedema. When a limb is affected, measurements may be taken to compare the size of the affected limb with that of the unaffected limb.

- **Pitting edema** is an early sign of lymphedema. *Pitting edema* is present when a swollen area is pressed and the pressure leaves a small indentation that slowly fills in again (Figure 2.1).

- **Stemmer's sign** is a thickened skin fold at the base of the second toe or finger that cannot be lifted when pinched.[1] (This fold is visible at the base of the toes in Figure 1-1.) This sign is positive in early primary lymphedema; however, it does not develop until later in cases of secondary lymphedema. A positive Stemmer's sign is an indication of lymphedema but a negative Stemmer's sign does not always exclude it.

Rule Outs

When lymphedema is suspected, the physician must first rule out any other conditions that might be causing the symptoms. A *rule-out* is the process of eliminating conditions that could possibly be causing the presenting symptoms. For example:

- **Sudden swelling** in the leg could be caused by a deep venous thrombosis. *Thrombosis* is the condition of having a blood clot attached to the wall of a blood vessel. This is a serious threat because the clot could break loose, travel through the bloodstream, and block a major artery in the lungs or brain.

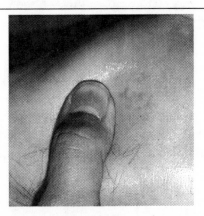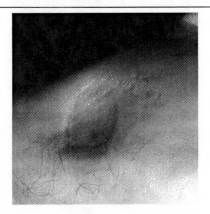

Figure 2-1: Testing for pitting edema using gentle pressure.

- **Slowly progressive swelling,** particularly of the legs, could be due to other conditions, such as chronic venous insufficiency, which impair the circulation. These conditions are discussed in Chapter 7.

- **Rapidly progressive and painful lymphedema-type swelling** could be due to a fast-growing tumor that places pressure on the lymph nodes. Although this condition is known as malignant lymphedema, the lymphedema itself is not cancerous. It is the tumor that is malignant.[2]

- **Lymphatic filariasis,** a tropical disease caused by a parasite.

Imaging Techniques

In cases where it is difficult to reach a diagnosis, imaging and more complex diagnostic testing may be necessary.

Lymphoscintigraphy, also known as *lymphangioscintigraphy*, is an imaging technique that involves the injection of a water-based contrast medium that does not damage the lymphatic tissues.[3] A *contrast medium* is a substance that is injected to make structures—such as lymphatic vessels—that otherwise would be difficult to see, more visible. In the past an oil-based contrast medium was used; this substance was damaging to the lymphatic tissues.

This radioactive contrast medium makes it possible for a gamma camera to trace the flow of lymph in the affected tissue. A computer then generates images based on the data gathered by the gamma camera.

When necessary, computerized tomography (CT), magnetic resonance imaging (MRI), and ultrasound techniques are used to image tissues and structures that cannot be seen effectively with lymphoscintigraphy.

The Stages of Lymphedema

Once lymphedema has been diagnosed, the physician or lymphedema therapist may identify the stage of this condition. *Staging* is a system used to

---

Stories of Lymph Notes Members

- I found my lymphedema after an airplane flight. Shame they don't warn us sooner. Might have been prevented. Tingling and numbness is not normal and needs checking on.

- I am 39 and have been taking water pills for "swelling" since I was 19. (I've had odd shaped legs since puberty.) I have struggled with weight all of my life, but when I got cellulitis for the second time in one year, I decided it was time to find out what was going on. I was just diagnosed with lymphedema.

- I have primary lymphedema in both legs and it is currently entering stage 2. This is complicated by the fact that I also have multiple sclerosis and lupus. At this point, I think the primary lymphedema is the most debilitating of all of these.

- I am a cervical cancer survivor 3 yrs. now. I have lymphedema of my left leg. It swells all the time but I am still here so it is a small price to pay.

---

describe the progression or severity of a disease. The three-part system described here is recommended by the International Society of Lymphology.[4]

Although lymphedema is a chronic condition, a patient who is receiving appropriate treatment will **not** necessarily progress from one stage to the next.

Stage 1 Lymphedema

In Stage 1 lymphedema the swollen tissues are soft to the touch and pitting edema is present. This swelling can be temporarily reduced by elevation of the limb; however, the swelling soon returns. Stage 1 lymphedema can be managed with early treatment and often improves greatly.

Stage 2 Lymphedema

In Stage 2 lymphedema tissues feel firm, even hard, and pressure leaves only a slight indentation. The tissue changes at this stage increase the risks of more swelling, fibrosis, infections, and skin problems. (*Fibrosis* is the formation of fine scar-like structures that cause the tissues to harden.) Stage 2 lymphedema usually can be improved with intense treatment.

Stage 3 Lymphedema

In Stage 3 lymphedema the swelling and tissue fibrosis cause the skin to harden and lose its normal elasticity. These changes create folds of tissue that limit mobility and are disfiguring. The creases within these folds encourage the formation of fungal infections and open wounds that are difficult to heal. Stage 3 lymphedema can be improved with intense therapy and it can be prevented from becoming worse; however, it is rarely reversed to an earlier stage. Figure 2-2 shows Stage 3 lymphedema in which the swelling of the legs has been reduced with treatment; however, hardened skin hanging in folds with deep creases is still present.

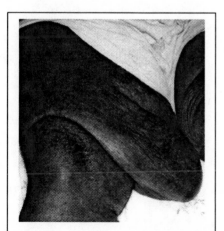

Figure 2-2: Stage 3 lymphedema after treatment has reduced the swelling. Excess folds of skin still remain.

Barbara's Story, Part II—Diagnosis

I head home to call my doctor for an appointment and my surgeon tells me to come right in. When he looks at my puffy hand—
the hand whose veins I used to hate, a work hand, a plain hand, a
bony hand—that now I would give anything to get back, he says,
yes, it looks like lymphedema and gives me the name of a physical
therapist who deals with this at a nearby treatment center. Meanwhile he tapes my hand and wrist.

I realize that everyone has a specialty, and those who might be
artists when it comes to carving cancer out of your breast might
not have a grip on taping your hand for lymphedema. By the time
I go out to dinner with the Bosom Buddies, the tips of my fingers
have turned blue.

All of us in the group share a crazed fear of the side effects of cancer and they understand the seriousness of getting lymphedema.
They also understand that it can't be a good thing to have blue
fingers, so they loosen the bandages for me.

continued on page 46

Chapter **3**

The Treatment of Lymphedema

An Overview of Lymphedema Treatment

Effective lymphedema treatment depends on close cooperation between the lymphedema therapist and the patient, and focuses on clearly stated treatment goals. This chapter includes an overview of lymphedema treatment techniques, compression methods, specialized treatment equipment, and ends with a discussion of treatment methods that do not work for lymphedema.

The Patient's First Visit

Prior to the first visit, a patient usually receives a written prescription from a healthcare provider referring him or her for lymphedema treatment. At the first visit, also known as the *intake interview*, the patient is asked to complete paperwork including a medical history and patient registration form.

During the interview the therapist will ask and answer questions, perform an examination of the affected area, and probably take measurements to be used as a baseline to evaluate the effectiveness of treatment.

If the patient's medical history includes other conditions that can impact the lymphedema treatment, the therapist will consult with the patient's physician before beginning any treatment. Often a new-patient orientation program is provided at this visit and the patient is scheduled for a series of appointments as needed.

New Patient Orientation

Because lymphedema treatment is based on the unique functioning of the lymphatic system, most new-patient orientation programs begin with an overview of the lymphatic system. In this book, essential information about the lymphatic system is provided in Section IV "Understanding the Lymphatic System."

To help the patient know what to expect during treatment, the orientation program includes an explanation of the components of lymphedema treatment and the role of the patient or caregiver in the self-management phase of treatment. In this book, the treatment phases are explained in this chapter and self-management is discussed in Section III "Self-Management of Lymphedema."

Treatment Phases

The treatment plan for each patient is designed to meet the patient's needs as determined at the intake interview and adapted based on ongoing evaluation. Treatment usually involves an intensive (see below) followed by an optimization phase. The intensive may be repeated periodically, if needed.

The Intensive

An intensive, also known as an *intervention*, is often required when a patient begins treatment. This consists of a series of daily visits for a period of one or more weeks. The goals of this treatment phase are to start reducing the swelling and to prepare the patient to continue and maintain this improvement.

Each visit during this treatment phase will typically include manual lymph drainage, bandaging, and training in self-management skills. By the end of the intensive, the patient should:

- See improvement in the affected area.

- Be equipped with appropriate compression aids.

- Have mastered self-management skills for use at home.

After the end of the intensive, the patient is usually seen for visits that are increasingly further apart. At each visit the patient is treated and the effectiveness of his or her self-management program is evaluated. When progress is satisfactory, the patient moves into the optimization phase.

The Optimization Phase

During the ongoing optimization phase, the patient is responsible for carrying out the self-management program on a daily basis. If there are questions or problems, a therapist is seen on an "as needed" basis. Routine follow-up visits are typically scheduled at six-month intervals to evaluate progress and verify that compression garments and aids still fit and function properly.

Due to a variety of factors related to their condition, not all patients are able to achieve this optimization stage. Regular ongoing professional treatments are necessary for these patients.

The Components of Lymphedema Treatment

The most widely accepted method of lymphedema treatment is known as *Complete Decongestive Therapy (CDT)*, *Complex Decongestive Therapy (CDT)*, or *Complete Decongestive Physiotherapy (CDP)*.

Although the names differ slightly, these treatment methods all use a combination of:

- Manual lymph drainage

- Compression techniques

- Self-management activities

Manual Lymph Drainage

Manual lymph drainage (MLD, which is pronounced M-L-D), is performed to stimulate the flow of lymph away from the affected area.[1] MLD is based on specialized manual techniques that have been used successfully in Europe since the 1930's. As shown in Figure 3-1, this is a gentle and pleasant treatment.

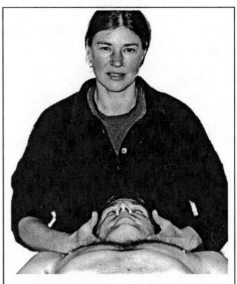

Figure 3-1: Manual Lymph Drainage begins with the neck region.

- **Light sweeping MLD movements** encourage the flow of lymph into the lymphatic capillaries located just under the skin.

- **Stronger MLD strokes** cause the lymph to flow into the lymphatic vessels deeper within the tissues.

- **Specialized stronger MLD** movements are also performed to soften hardened (fibrotic) tissues.

The MLD portion of the treatment session usually lasts from 30 to 60 minutes, depending on the size of the affected area(s), the severity of the symptoms, and the amount of fibrosis.[2]

It is important that the patient drink plenty of water after an MLD session to replenish the fluids that were mobilized by this treatment. The patient can expect an increased need to urinate soon after a treatment and for several hours thereafter. This occurs as the excess fluid which was removed from the tissues is processed by the kidneys and excreted as urine.

Between professional visits a type of MLD, known as self-massage, is performed by the patient or caregiver as part of the self-management program (see Chapter 10).

Contraindications for Manual Lymph Drainage

MLD *should not* be performed if any of the following conditions are present or are suspected:[3]

☐ Cellulitis or any other acute infection.

☐ Fever or any other indication of a developing infection.

☐ Any other major health problems that are not under control, unless treatment has been approved by the patient's physician.

If potential contraindications are present, the therapist may consult the patient's physician before providing MLD treatment.

Compression Goals

Specialized forms of compression are essential elements of lymphedema treatment. Compression is used to:

- Maintain the progress made in reducing swelling during the MLD treatment.

- Prevent or minimize additional swelling.

- Support the natural drainage of lymph from the tissues.

- Provide resistance that enhances the effectiveness of muscle movements in stimulating the flow of lymph. *Resistance* is added pressure created when muscle movement presses against the garment or bandage.

- Aid in softening fibrotic tissues.

Compression Methods Compared

Bandages are an effective and flexible form of compression for use when the patient is active or resting (see Figures 3-2 and 3-4).

Compression garments are knit two-way stretch sleeves or stockings worn during the day to assist in controlling swelling and to aid in moving lymph from the affected area (see Figure 3-3).

Compression aids are custom-fitted sleeves, stockings, or pads that are worn when the patient is active or resting. Compression aids help to control swelling, enhance the flow of lymph, and assist in softening fibrotic tissues (see Figure 3-4).

Stories of Lymph Notes Members

Having been diagnosed with primary lymphedema in 1989, I had already spent two years where doctors were confused, concerned and really did not know which way to turn. In hospital, at one midnight, I was told to make my peace with God and my family because I would not be alive the following morning. Very scary and sobering to say the least.

Three specialists were present: one in internal medicine, one in infectious diseases, and the third a skin doctor. Everything they tried provided very temporary relief. When one of them learned of a physiotherapist who had recently studied the treatment of lymphedema through gentle pressure and two way stretch bandages, my world improved in leaps and bounds. My weight went down over fifty pounds in my legs alone. Now, 16 years later, I still take low dosage penicillin twice daily and wear compression stockings reverting to bandages every two or three weeks for one day.

Life has returned to a very active one and is beautiful.

Stories of Lymph Notes Members

I was born with lymphedema of my right hand and arm 67 years ago. Although very sympathetic, my doctors were not very much help. Mainly they told me that I should be thankful that I can use the arm and hand and that I should learn to live with the lymphedema.

About 8 years ago, I read in a magazine that there was massage therapy available to treat lymphedema. I made many inquiries and finally underwent six weeks of therapy. The results even amazed my doctor and my therapist. The size of my arm decreased greatly. Though not as slender as the other arm, it is fine as it is because it feels so much lighter. My shoulder is less droopy from the weight, and for the first time in my life, I am able to buy readymade clothes without having the sleeves altered. I am thankful to say that the reduction has been maintained, with the help of compression garments.

Bandages

Bandages are effective because they can:

- Accommodate the changing size of a limb as it decreases in size.

- Provide pressure to continue the reduction of the swollen limb.

- Control additional swelling.

- Soften fibrotic tissues. *Fibrotic* means pertaining to abnormally hardened tissues.

- Create working pressure to move lymph during exercise. *Working pressure* is caused by the motion of muscles in the bandaged limb while walking or exercising.

- Increase resistance during activity.

- Be flexible enough to be worn 23 hours a day.

Bandaging During an Intensive

During the intensive phase of treatment, bandages are worn constantly, 23 hours a day for seven days a week (Figure 3-2). For a short time each day the bandages are removed so the patient can bathe or shower before fresh bandages are placed. Between visits, and while bandaged, the patient is expected to exercise and remain active.

After the intensive phase, if the patient still requires the level of compression provided by bandages, self-bandaging becomes part of the self-management program as explained in Chapter 11.

Compression Garments

Compression garments are specialized elastic knit two-way stretch sleeves or stockings that can be worn under clothing throughout the day, including while exercising.

Compression garments are *not worn* while sleeping because they provide too much compression when the body is inactive. Also, if the garment moves out of place during sleep, it could cause constriction that damages the circulation.

Compression garments do not provide protection against sunburn and, unless an outer layer of clothing is worn, a high SPF sunscreen should be applied under the compression garment.

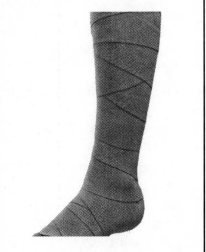

Figure 3-2: Bandages provide effective compression.

Compression Sleeves

When the arm is affected, a compression sleeve that covers the entire arm from the wrist to the shoulder is worn. Wearing a compression sleeve just to the elbow is usually not recommended. When the hand is also affected, a gauntlet (without finger coverage), or glove (with finger coverage), may be worn in addition to a sleeve.

Compression Stockings

When one leg is involved, a single stocking is worn. When both legs are involved, either a pair of stockings or a single pantyhose-style garment is worn. Compression stockings often leave the toes exposed to avoid pressure points or the formation of calluses.

Fitting of Compression Garments

• Compression garments are custom measured for size so that the garment stays comfortably in place and fits smoothly without wrinkles or bulges that can damage the tissues (see Figure 3-3).

• Measurements for these garments should be taken by a trained fitter and the fit should be re-evaluated every six months. Garments that no longer fit properly should be replaced immediately.

• Compression garments are prescribed to provide the correct amount of pressure to enhance the control of swelling. Too little compression is ineffective and too much compression can damage the tissues.

Putting on Compression garments

At first, putting on a compression garment may seem difficult but with practice the process goes more smoothly. In addition to the suggestions provided here, most garment manufacturers provide helpful guides and some sell devices (called donning aids) to make this process easier.

Applying a low pH moisturizer to the affected limb is an important part of skin care. However, freshly applied moisturizer makes it more difficult to put on these garments. Instead of moisturizing just before putting on the garment in the morning, apply moisturizer in the evening after the garment has been removed.

- A compression garment is easier to put on early in the day before swelling occurs.

- Apply a thin layer of cornstarch or powder over your carefully dried skin to help the garment slide more easily.

- Do not wear rings or jewelry that can snag and damage your garment.

- Wearing rubber or vinyl gloves while putting on the garment provides a better grip on the fabric and prevents fingernails from damaging the fabric.

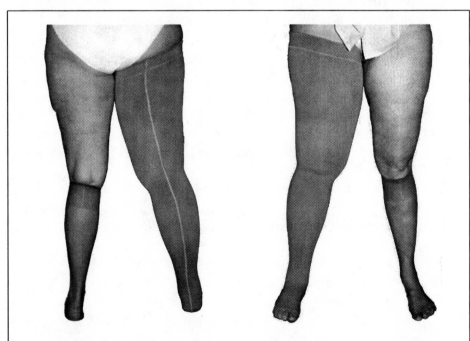

Figure 3-3: Properly fitting compression garments are worn during the day.

When the garment is in place it should fit smoothly without wrinkles or bunched areas that can irritate the tissues.

Care of Compression Garments

Ideally the patient should have two of each compression garments: so they have one to wear while the other one is being cleaned. These garments should be hand-laundered following the manufacturer's instructions. The specialized liquid soaps sold by the garment manufacturers are designed to thoroughly clean the garment and to enhance the durability of the garment's elastic. Compression garments should be placed flat to dry.

Compression Aids

The term *compression aid* describes a variety of custom-fitted garments or pads that consist of a layer of foam padding stitched between covers of a specialized fabric in a channel-like pattern to stimulate the flow of lymph.

- The design of these products produces differing pressures on the limb.

- The channeling pattern of the stitching may assist in directing the flow of lymph into alternate pathways around the obstructed area.

- A lymphedema therapist usually recommends the appropriate type of compression aid and does the fitting.

- Unlike compression garments, compression aids can be worn during the day and night.

- Compression aids are **not** worn with compression garments.

Contour Garments

Contour garments are compression aids that cover the entire affected arm or leg. Some styles utilize straps and Velcro® fasteners to provide precise pressure as needed along the limb. Other styles use less complex fasteners and are less bulky, cooler, and are donned more easily.

When limited additional compression is required, a tight outer layer known as a "power sleeve" is worn over the compression garment. For greater compression, the patient can bandage directly over the contour garment (Figure 3-4).

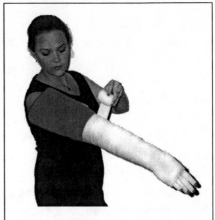

Figure 3-4: A compression aid is worn when the patient is active or resting. For increased compression, bandages may be placed directly over the compression aid.

Contour Pads

Contour pads are compression aids used primarily in treating lymphedema of the trunk. For example, after a single mastectomy a compression pad that wraps from the midline in the front to the midline in the back of the affected side is worn to control swelling and to soften fibrotic tissue. The pad is usually held firmly in place by a sports bra that opens in the front.

The Pump

At one time, "the pump" was the only available form of lymphedema therapy. Initially these treatments were so painful that they were administered under general anesthesia and some pump treatments were more damaging than they were helpful.

A new generation of pumps, known as *sequential gradient compression pumps* or *pneumatic pumps,* is now available. This pump consists of a garment that encases the affected limb and automatically pushes air into channels built into the garment (Figure 3-5). The controls on the pump cause the garment to gently inflate and release in sequential movements designed to imitate the natural flow of lymph. Normally this flow would be due to the smooth muscle contractions in the lymphatic vessels and by the movements of nearby muscles and blood vessels.

The acceptance of the pump as the preferred form of lymphedema treatment has declined sharply since the early 1990's when Complete Decongestive Therapy (CDT) was proven to be more effective. Also, recent research indicates that the use of the pump can increase fibrosis and displace the swelling of the limb toward the body and into the trunk or genitalia.[4]

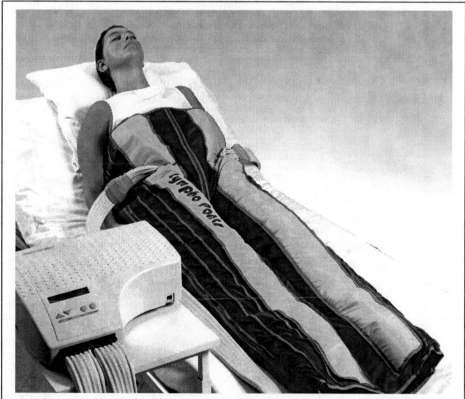

Figure 3-5: A sequential pneumatic pump in use to treat edema of the legs

The Pump During Professional Care

Despite its limitations, a pump can successfully be incorporated into professional lymphedema treatment when these protocols are followed:

1. The therapist must see and evaluate the patient first.

2. Before the pump is used, manual lymph drainage must be performed on the neck, abdomen, and the uninvolved leg or arm. This prepares the lymphatic system to receive the fluid that the pump will remove from the affected arm or leg.

   If MLD is not performed, the pump may squeeze fluid from the affected leg or arm into the area adjacent to the sleeve where it may not move into the body as it should. When the arm is involved, having fluid pushed into the body can cause lymphedema of the chest wall. When the leg is involved, having fluid pushed into the body can cause genital lymphedema.

3. The patient's ongoing progress must be monitored carefully with emphasis on looking for any indications of fibrosis or increasing swelling in surrounding tissues.

Use of the Pump at Home

Patients who have difficulty getting to a therapist, or who lack insurance coverage for professional treatment, may be interested in having a pump for home care. This option is made more appealing when the pump is classified as durable medical equipment (DME) that Medicare and other insurance plans will help pay for.

- **Learning to use the pump at home.** Before starting a program of pump use at home, it is very important that a therapist train the patient or caregiver to use it properly. This includes instruction in how to set the pump's pressure levels and which pressure levels to use. The therapist should periodically examine the patient's limbs to evaluate his or her condition in response to the use of the pump.

- **Advance preparation.** Before beginning a pump session, it is necessary to examine the limb for any signs of infection or breaks in the skin. The pump should not be used when an infection is present.

- **Self-Massage is essential.** The requirements for MLD before beginning a pump treatment are the same at home as they are in a treatment facility. The difference is that it is the patient, or caregiver, who performs the self-massage before the home treatment. Self-massage is discussed in Chapter 10.

- **Treatment session length.** Manufacturers usually recommend using the pump from one to four hours daily, preferably in the evening. If necessary, this can be divided into two sessions with half in the morning and half in the evening.

- **After the treatment.** Self-massage is performed again after the pump treatment. The purpose of this self-massage is to move the lymph from where the pump ends upwards to the terminus.

Chest Wall Lymphedema

Chest wall lymphedema, also known as *truncal lymphedema*, may develop in conjunction with arm and hand lymphedema following breast cancer treatment.[5] This type of lymphedema affects the armpit, shoulder joint, back, and chest wall.

Symptoms include widespread swelling, tingling, joint discomfort, and pain. Women who have been treated for breast cancer and find wearing a prosthesis or bra to be painful may have developed chest wall lymphedema.

Treatment of Chest Wall Lymphedema

Manual lymph drainage is very important in removing excess fluid and softening fibrotic tissues in this area. A patient with chest wall lymphedema often requires frequent visits for MLD.

Compression is important in treating lymphedema, but effective compression of the chest area is difficult to achieve. Specialized bras are available and feature adjustments to accommodate changes in chest dimension and to increase comfort. These bras provide some compression and include a prosthesis pocket and additional pockets to hold compression aids when needed.

Compression aids such as foam chip pads or custom fitted quilted garments are used to soften fibrotic tissue and to provide compression in this area.

Bandaging is of limited value on the chest area for two reasons: First, bandages are designed to work with the pumping action of muscles and this kind of muscle action is not present in the chest. Second, because of the constant changes in chest size while breathing, it is difficult to bandage effectively and to keep these bandages in place.

Self-massage is particularly important in the chest region because compression methods alone cannot control the swelling. Self-massage is explained in Chapter 10.

Daily exercise, which includes walking and arm exercises, is also important in stimulating the flow of lymph and in maintaining mobility of the affected arm and shoulder. Swimming and water exercise are also beneficial in treating chest lymphedema (see Chapter 13).

Kinesio Tape®

Kinesio tape, which looks like wide adhesive tape, was originally designed to treat sports injuries and has proven to be a versatile tool that is beneficial in treating a wide range of conditions including lymphedema affecting the chest and arm (Figure 3-6).[6]

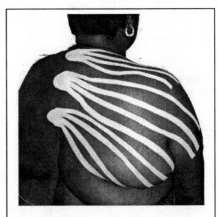

Figure 3-6: Kinesio tape as shown here, is being used to stimulate the flow of lymph across the back.

Because the effectiveness of Kinesio tape depends on its correct placement, only lymphedema therapists with this specialized training should perform Kinesio taping.

Kinesio Tape Details

This tape is made of 100 percent high-grade cotton that is latex-free. An average application will stay in place for three to four days and can be worn while swimming or showering. The backing of the tape is covered with a very light, heat-activated, adhesive applied in small wave-like channels.

The thickness and elasticity of the tape is similar to that of the outer layer of the skin. Since the tape has the same flexibility as human skin, the tape does not bind or restrict circulation even on swollen tissues.

According to the manufacturer, Kinesio tape is beneficial in lymphedema treatment because:

- The channels carry sweat and water away from the skin and encourage the flow of lymph.

- The tape backing gently lifts the skin in the wave-like channel pattern. This lifting action helps to take pressure off the interstitial fluid just below the skin and allows for greater lymph drainage.

- As the body moves, the tape acts like a pump, continually stimulating the circulation of lymph.

Treatments That Do Not Work For Lymphedema

There are some traditional medical treatments for swelling that *are not* effective in the treatment of lymphedema. Your lymphedema therapist will not suggest these treatments but concerned family, friends, or a poorly informed healthcare provider might. It is in your best interest to understand *why* these treatments are not beneficial for lymphedema.

Diuretics

Diuretics, often referred to as *water pills*, are frequently prescribed when swelling is present due to a heart condition or similar cause. These pills work by stimulating the kidneys to remove more fluid from the bloodstream.

Since lymphedema also involves swelling, a commonly asked question is, *"What about diuretics? Won't they work for lymphedema too?"* The swelling of lymphedema is caused by damage to the lymphatic system that traps this fluid in the tissues. Stimulating the kidneys will not reduce this swelling. For this reason, diuretics are not a recommended treatment for lymphedema.

However, a patient with lymphedema who also has hypertension, or any of the other conditions that are normally treated with diuretics, may safely take these medications when they are prescribed to treat these other conditions.

Taping to Control Swelling

There have been reported cases of physicians and other healthcare providers who advise wrapping a limb with adhesive tape in an effort to prevent further lymphedema swelling. This type of tape cannot prevent further swelling and this tape does not expand as the swelling increases. As illustrated by Barbara's and Megan's stories, this can be uncomfortable and dangerous if the tape cuts off the circulation in the affected area.

Ace Bandages

Ace bandages, also known as *long-stretch bandages,* are useful for the support and relief of sprains and dislocations. These bandages have also been tried in the treatment of lymphedema but they are not effective for routine use.

Long-stretch bandages expand up to about 180 percent. This amount of stretch *does not* support the efforts of the working muscles. In contrast, the short-stretch bandages used in treating lymphedema expand only up to 70 percent and provide resistance that supports and enhances the pumping motion of the muscles. This resistance aids in the upward flow of lymph.

Megan's Story

During the summer of Megan's fourteenth birthday a bee stung her on her right foot. The swelling wasn't serious but it continued for several weeks and into the beginning of soccer season. Because her foot was still swollen, Megan saw her pediatrician and he carefully wrapped the ankle to control the swelling.

By the next morning, Megan's entire leg was swollen. Right away her Mother knew what was wrong. Several years before, Megan's grandmother had experienced similar swelling and had been diagnosed as having primary lymphedema. Despite the family history, it took visits to several different doctors to get an "official diagnosis."

Happily Megan is now being treated by a qualified therapist, has learned the necessary self-management skills, and is on her way to living well with lymphedema.

The exception to the use of Ace bandages is for patients who are nonambulatory. *Ambulatory* means able to walk, *nonambulatory* means unable to walk. For nonambulatory patients, long-stretch bandages can help to control swelling without providing the unneeded resistance of short-stretch bandages.

Applying Heat

With swelling due to an injury, the traditional treatment includes applying cold to the area for the first 24 hours and then changing to hot packs in ongoing efforts to control the swelling. Cold packs will not decrease the swelling of lymphedema and applying hot packs will make the swelling worse!

Barbara's Story, Part III—Treatment

Now I'm afraid I'll look like elephant lady at the altar. How will R. put the silver wedding band on my sausage finger? "I've got to have my arm and hand back to normal in eight weeks," I tell the physical therapist. "I'm getting married."

She's realistic and up front, no sugarcoating about this. Lymphedema can more than triple of the size of your arm, she tells me. With treatment I may or may not get the current swelling down, and if I do, I'll always have to take special precautions. When I fly, I'll have to wear a special sleeve and glove. This is a chronic disease and may or may not come back no matter what I do.

In the meantime, my hand and arm will be bandaged, and I'll have special massages, special exercises. She shows me the way to tape my hand and fingers. It will take me days to learn how to do this properly. The good news is that your fingers don't turn blue when it's done right.

Twice a week now I have treatment for lymphedema -- a drainage massage, which sounds like an awful plumbing procedure, but is in fact quite pleasant; nothing you can see actually drains. Meanwhile, I wear the bandages wrapped all the way up to my armpit. When they see my bandaged hand and arm, strangers ask me what happened. Sometimes I tell them I fell off a horse, it was a skydiving accident, or it happened when I was surfing. I've become the Walter Mitty of risky sports.

Gradually the swelling comes down. My arm and hand have miraculously returned to normal, but I keep the bandages on to be sure.

continued on page 56

Chapter **4**

Finding Quality
Lymphedema Treatment

Unless the referring healthcare provider recommends a specific treatment center or therapist, it is up to the patient and their family to select a treatment center and therapist. This chapter covers:

- Training standards for lymphedema therapists.

- Tips on locating and selecting treatment centers and therapists.

- Suggestions for what to do if treatment is not helping.

- Options for situations where treatment is not available.

Lymphedema Therapist Training

Lymphedema therapy is a specialized skill that requires a deep understanding of the physiology of the lymphatic system combined with hands-on massage skills. Manual lymph drainage is different from the 'lymphatic massage' offered by aestheticians and non-medical massage therapists.

The National Lymphedema Network created the Lymphology Association of North America (LANA) in 2001 to establish training standards for lymphedema therapists and to create a national program to certify qualified therapists.[1]

CLT-LANA Training

The LANA standards for a Certified Lymphedema Therapist (CLT-LANA) require 135 hours of specialized education in the treatment of lymphedema including one-third theoretical instruction in the anatomy and physiology of the lymphatic system, and two-thirds hands-on mentored training.

The prerequisite for this training is professional license as a physical therapist (PT), physical therapy assistant (PTA), occupational therapist (OT), occupational therapy assistant (OTA), registered nurse (RN), physician (MD), physician's assistant (PA) licensed athletic trainer (ATL), or a licensed massage therapist (LMT) with 500 massage school hours and/or a National Therapeutic Massage and Bodywork Certification plus 12 hours of college level anatomy and physiology.

Programs offering LANA standard training are listed on the next page.

LANA Certification

The professional title CLT-LANA (Certified Lymphedema Therapist-LANA) is bestowed upon therapists that have completed a training program meeting the LANA standards, have one or more years of work experience in the field, and have passed the written LANA Certification Test.

The LANA certificate must be renewed every six years either by re-examination or by documenting continuing education credits.

Therapists Who Are Not LANA Certified

LANA certification is a voluntary and relatively new program. There are many qualified therapists who have met the LANA training requirements but have not yet elected to take part in the examination program.

Whether or not a therapist is LANA certified, it is important to determine that he or she has completed specialized lymphedema training that meets the LANA requirements.

LANA Standard Training Programs

Academy of Lymphatic Studies   www.acols.com

Dr. Vodder School of North America   www.vodderschool.com

Klose Training and Consulting   www.klosetraining.com

Norton School of Lymphatic Therapy   www.nortonschool.com

The Upledger Institute   www.upledger.com

Locating a Treatment Center/Therapist

Many hospitals provide lymphedema treatment as an outpatient program through the rehabilitation, physical therapy, occupational therapy department, or breast cancer rehabilitation program. Other potential settings for lymphedema treatment include some rehabilitation centers, physical therapy practices, specialized lymphedema treatment facilities, and lymphedema therapists in private practice.

These resources may help you locate a therapist or center:

- Ask your insurance company, preferred provider organization, or HMO about therapists within their network.

- Lymph Notes (www.lymphnotes.com) provides a directory of lymphedema treatment facilities and lymphedema support groups.

- The National Lymphedema Network resource guide includes information on facilities and therapists (www.lymphnet.org).

- The LANA web site (www.clt-lana.org) includes a list, by state, of therapists who have passed this examination.

- Each of the training programs listed above publishes a list of graduates on their web site. If you find a listing for a therapist that shows only a telephone number, try searching online for the telephone number; frequently the search results will include the facility where the therapist is (or was) employed.

- Look in the telephone directory under Physical Therapy.

- Call hospitals in your area and ask if they provide lymphedema treatment. Try the physical therapy, occupational therapy, rehabilitation services, and oncology departments.

- Locate cancer support groups (look at www.cancer.org and in the telephone book under Cancer Education, Referral and Support), undoubtedly at least one person in the group will have lymphedema.

Screening Questions for Centers/Therapists

Copy the list of questions on the next page, add your own questions, and use the answers to help you screen treatment centers and therapists. Hopefully you will get the following answers:

1. **What training do your therapists have?**
   Therapists should have training that meets the LANA standard and, ideally, LANA certification.

2. **What treatment methods do you use?**
   Complete Decongestive Therapy (CDT), manual lymph drainage (MLD), compression, and self-management techniques are the most widely accepted forms of lymphedema treatment.

3. **Is 'the pump' routinely used in treatment sessions?**
   The pump is no longer widely accepted as part of routine treatments. If the pump is used, it should always be in conjunction with Complete Decongestive Therapy performed by a qualified therapist.

4. **Will your therapists teach me, or my caregiver, how to perform self-massage and other self-management skills?**
   Self-management is an important part of treating lymphedema and

Therapist/Treatment Center Questions

Center: _____

Therapist: _____

Date: _____

1. What training do you/your therapists have?

   _____

   _____

2. What treatment methods do you/your therapists use?

   _____

   _____

3. Is 'the pump' routinely used in treatment?

   _____

4. Will you/your therapists teach me, or my caregiver, how to perform self-massage and other self-management skills?

   _____

   _____

Notes: _____

   _____

you need to learn these skills as they apply to your condition. Once you have learned these techniques, it is your responsibility to follow through on them at home.

When Treatment is Not Helping

As shown in the table below, there are clear indications when lymphedema treatment is or is not helping.

Is Lymphedema Treatment Successful?	
Treatment is Successful When...	**Treatment is Not Helping When...**
Swelling decreases	Swelling increases
Tissues remain soft	Tissues become hard (fibrotic)
Infections occur less often	Infections are more frequent
Quality of life improves	Quality of life is deteriorating

Doing nothing may not be a good option when treatment is not helping. If the therapist does not initiate changes in the treatment, it is up to the patient and their family to take action so that he or she receives adequate treatment.

The first step toward finding a solution is identifying the problem. Only then is it possible to make the appropriate changes. Since treatment consists of self-management and professional care, identifying the problem must examine both of these components.[2]

Self-Management

Start with an honest evaluation by the patient, or caregiver, of how regularly and completely the self-management program is being carried out between treatments:

☐ Are you performing appropriate skin care as part of your daily routine?

☐ Do you wear your compression garments regularly and properly?

☐ Are you performing self-massage as prescribed?

☐ Do you complete your exercise program regularly?

If compliance in self-management is a problem, it may be necessary to obtain additional training in these skills or to seek help in maintaining the motivation necessary to manage your program successfully. See Section III "Self-Management of Lymphedema."

Professional Care

If self-management is being implemented properly but the lymphedema is not responding, it is necessary to have your condition reevaluated to determine if changes in your medical condition are causing the problems being experienced.

Stories of Lymph Notes Members

I am 40 years old and I have lymphedema in my right hand and wrist from breast surgery 13 years ago. I underwent treatment and found it more annoying than helpful. I have not had any treatment for years and I battle constant swelling and pain. I would like to find some help. I am afraid that letting this go will only make the swelling worse. Help!

If there are no changes in your condition to account for the lack of progress, you should consult with the director of the clinic about changing to a different therapist. Therapists can vary in their approach and sometimes a patient-therapist combination does not work as well as it should.

If you do not get satisfactory answers from the clinic director, or do not begin to show progress, it may be time to change to a different treatment facility.

What to do When Treatment is Not Readily Available

There are so many reasons why individuals find it difficult, if not impossible, to receive proper lymphedema treatment. These include the shortage of qualified therapists, not living near a treatment facility, and financial issues. If you are in such a situation, the following suggestions can help you find a good solution.

Learn All You Can About Lymphedema

Reading this book is an excellent beginning. The more you know, the better prepared you are to be your own advocate. Pay special attention to the steps described in Section III "Self-Management of Lymphedema." Once you have been taught these techniques by a therapist, you should be able to better control your condition at home by carefully performing the steps in your self-management program.

When Money is the Issue

If finances are preventing you from getting treatment, contact the hospital social worker or your local social services to see what aid may be available. Dealing with insurance plans is discussed in Chapter 5.

Stories of Lymph Notes Members

I was born in 1926 and had erysipelas [see page 77] several times before the age of six. We lived in Oklahoma and the doctor was miles away in another town so my father cared for me by administering epsom salt soaks and applying ointments. At age 10, I had a very high fever and pneumonia. A result of this illness was swelling in my right ankle.

All of this happened before sulfa drugs and penicillin were available, so my doctor used a mustard plaster and an oxygen tent. At age 20, my left ankle and leg began swelling.

I have now lived 78+ years with lymphedema. My doctors still have little or no knowledge of the condition. I am so thankful that information is finally coming out.

The Trip Too Far

If you find a treatment center, but it is too distant for frequent treatments to be practical, make every effort to schedule at least one or two visits.

- Prepare for these visits by creating a list of questions you need answered (see Chapter 15).

- Explain your travel problem to the therapist and ask if it would be possible to teach you self-management skills for use at home until you are able to begin a full treatment program.

- Ask if it would be acceptable to have someone (friend, caregiver, family member) come with you to video tape these instructions.

Barbara's Story, Part IV—The Wedding

In the same chapel where I sent up prayers for courage exactly six months ago when I was diagnosed with breast cancer, I now walk down the aisle on my brother's arm, toward R., waiting for me at the altar with our five children standing on either side of him. The pews are filled with our extended family and close friends. The chapel is lit with candles and filled with white flowers. The organist plays "Sheep May Safely Graze" and all around me are the faces of people I love.

The marriage vows take on a whole new meaning as R. and I repeat them to one another. Here is a man who never blinked when he learned I had breast cancer, who would take me with or without breasts, and with an arm and hand that could look like a pincushion at any instant.

Chapter 5

Insurance and Reimbursement Issues

Just as lymphedema treatment and self management are essential to your physical health, reimbursement and record keeping may be essential to your financial health. America may or may not have the most advanced health-care system but we certainly have the most complicated health insurance system. A complete guide to health care reimbursement could fill an entire book and would be out of date before it could be printed.

Unfortunately the insurance industry has been slow in understanding lymph-edema, recognizing the value of currently accepted lymphedema treatments, and appreciating the risks and costs of not treating lymphedema. Obtaining insurance reimbursement is often an added hurdle to overcome.

Clarify insurance coverage before starting treatment to minimize misunder-standings. Many lymphedema treatment facilities have a specialist who can assist with insurance issues.

Our brief guide to navigating this swamp is organized by topic to help you find the information that applies to your situation:

- Understanding Health Insurance Coverage

- Maximizing Reimbursement

- When Treatment is Denied

- Changing Insurance Plans

- Care Without Coverage

- Relevant Laws covering health insurance portability, accommodation for disabilities, medical leave, and post breast cancer coverage.

Understanding Health Insurance Coverage

Health insurance reimbursement is controlled by rules that define what types of treatment, equipment, or medication the insurance will cover for a given diagnosis. Coverage rules may be explained in plan documents including the Summary Plan Description (SPD), a Summary of Material Modifications (SMM), or a Summary Annual Report (SAR).

Coverage rules may change over time as companies respond to new legislation (see Relevant Laws below) and case law, new research on effectiveness and medical necessity, changes adopted by competitors and Medicare, and public pressure. Insurance companies are not required to provide advanced notice of changes in reimbursement rules.

What is Not Usually Covered

Many policies place limitations on their coverage of lymphedema treatment. It is not unusual for a policy to refuse to pay for:

- More than one treatment per day on an outpatient basis, even if the treatment plan recommends multiple daily visits during the intensive phase.

- Compression garments of any type including sleeves or stockings, or compression aids such as a Reid sleeve. These decisions can be appealed and are occasionally overturned.

- Bandages for use at home. Despite the fact that they are medically necessary, lymphedema bandages are rarely covered by insurance because they are considered to be disposable items for personal use.

- More than a fixed annual dollar amount for lymphedema treatment.

For suggestions on handling unreimbursed expenses see "Care Without Coverage" on page 67.

The Pump

Medicare, and many insurance companies, will pay part of the cost of a pump for use at home. If you are considering requesting a pump, it is important to clarify what steps you must take in order to qualify. Also identify how much of the cost will be your responsibility.

Having a pump at home does not replace your need for professional lymphedema treatment. Before deciding to get a pump, it is best to clarify that your additional treatment is still covered. If coverage for ongoing treatment is refused, you have the right to appeal that decision.

Maximizing Reimbursement

Good record keeping and persistence are the keys to reimbursement:

- Prepare accurate claims using the tips provided below.

- Track every reimbursement request you submit. Match payments with requests and follow-up on payments that are delayed.

- Take names, dates, and notes when you call the insurance company. Be assertive but remain polite.

- Create a paper trail by submitting requests in writing and confirming phone conversations. This demonstrates that you are serious and provides the documentation necessary for possible lobbying efforts or legal actions.

- If you have access to a fax machine, use it. Fax is faster than postal mail and acceptable as a legal record in many cases.

- If you use e-mail to correspond with your insurance company, keep printed copies of the messages you send and receive.

Preparing Accurate Claims

For faster processing, be sure your claims have the correct identifying information, diagnostic code, and treatment code as explained below.

Identifying Information

Verify that the identifying information on the claims is correct and legible. Depending on the form, this may include:

☐ Patient identification: name, medical record number, insurance identification number, group number.

☐ Insured party: name, insurance identification number, group number.

☐ Employer information: name, group number.

☐ Provider: name, title, license number, insurance identification number.

Insurance Claim Coding

Each healthcare insurance claim contains two codes that must match. One is the diagnostic code that identifies the disease or condition. The other code identifies the treatment provided. The treatment must be "appropriate" for the disease identified by the diagnostic code.

Diagnostic Codes

The International Classification of Diseases-9th Revision Clinical Modification (ICD-9 or ICD-9CM) is the coding system used to identify the disease or condition for which the patient is being treated. These codes are precise and must be entered correctly. For example, post-mastectomy lymphedema (457.0), secondary lymphedema due to other causes (457.1), primary lymphedema (757.0), and filariasis each have different codes.

You will find the ICD-9 code number on the check-out form you received at the end of your office visit. The same ICD-9 number should appear on the Explanation of Benefits (EOB) you receive from your insurance company.

Treatment Codes

The Current Procedural Terminology (CPT) is the coding system used to tell the insurance company what treatment you received at each visit. The treatment code must relate directly to the condition identified by the ICD-9 code on your claim. If you think there has been a coding error, ask the insurance clerk at your treatment center to check this information for you.

When Treatment Is Denied

The primary reasons why insurance companies deny coverage for lymphedema treatment are:

- Cost-containment measures that play a major role in insurance decisions today.

- Coding errors in preparing a claim or missing documentation. Review the Preparing Accurate Claims section above and resubmit your claim. Keep a copy in your files of this claim and any letter that accompanied it.

- A lack of understanding about lymphedema by those who review claims.

Letter of Appeal Checklist

☐ **Heading:** Your name, address, and telephone number.

☐ **Date:** This is the date when the letter was written.

☐ **Inside Address:** Name and address of the person in the appeals department of the insurance company.

☐ **Patient:** The patient's name, identification number, and group number.

☐ **Insured (if different):** The insured person's name, identification number, group number, and employer.

☐ **RE:** Appeal of Denial of Coverage letter dated <<*insert date* >> <<*reference number*>>

☐ **Greeting:** This is traditional—but increasingly optional.

☐ **Body:** Present your case here. Keep it brief, to the point, and business-like. You may incorporate our suggested wording.

☐ **Closing:** State your request (reconsideration of the denial, approval, etc.) and that you anticipate a prompt reply. "Thank you for your prompt attention" is always a nice touch.

☐ **Signature:** Your signature above your printed name.

☐ **Enclosures:** A list of enclosed documents identified by title and date. Include the prescription for lymphedema treatment, a copy of the letter of denial, and other relevant documents.

☐ **CC:** A list of names, titles, and addresses for those who are receiving copies of this letter.

Writing a Letter of Appeal

When a request for treatment is denied, the patient or the insured has the right to appeal, and should do so! Use the checklist on page 62 and the wording suggested below to:

- Clarify that this is a physician ordered treatment.

- Explain lymphedema, if necessary.

- Cite the Women's Health and Cancer Rights Act (WHCRA), if applicable.

Although it is tempting to telephone or send an e-mail, it is prudent to document any appeal in writing. Be sure to keep a copy of the letter in your files. If you do not receive a response in a timely manner, follow-up with a phone call (and letter) to the individual to whom you addressed your letter. Four weeks is considered to be a timely response.

The topics below provide suggested wording that can be used in a letter of appeal. Change the words shown in <<*brackets*>> to fit your situation.

Physician-Ordered Treatment

A patient seeking lymphedema treatment must have a prescription from his or her physician. If the insurance company denies or limits treatment, this is a refusal to cover physician-ordered treatment. The following is suggested wording for mentioning this factor:

> On <<*date of diagnosis*>>, Dr. <<*name of doctor*>> diagnosed lymphedema in my <<*list of affected body parts*>> as a result of <<*cause of lymphedema*>>. Lymphedema is a chronic condition requiring ongoing treatment administered by a qualified lymphedema therapist. A copy of the prescription ordering this treatment is enclosed.

Without this medically necessary treatment, <<*my/his/her*>> condition may become progressively worse with increasing pain, swelling, tissue deterioration (fibrosis, hyperkeratosis, papillomatosis) that often results in open wounds and infections (cellulitis, lymphangitis, erysipelas) that may require hospitalization. Untreated lymphedema can result in the loss of mobility and potentially total disability.

Explain Lymphedema

An expensive error on the part of many insurance companies is their failure to understand lymphedema. They do not recognize that lymphedema is a serious chronic condition that becomes progressively worse without treatment. They are not aware that the longer lymphedema is allowed to progress, the more expensive it will be to treat the lymphedema and its complications.

You can explain this condition clearly and authoritatively by quoting the following description:

> Lymphedema is a chronic condition that requires ongoing treatment as explained by the following statement from The Diagnosis and Treatment of Peripheral Lymphedema: Consensus Document of the International Society of Lymphology' *Lymphology* 23 (2003) 84-91: "*Because lymphedema is a chronic, generally incurable ailment, it requires as do other chronic disorders, lifelong care and attention along with psychosocial support. The continued need for therapy does not mean that treatment is unsatisfactory… For example patients with diabetes mellitus continue to need insulin or a special diet. Similarly, patients with lymphedema require lifelong care.*"

Mention the Women's Health and Cancer Rights Act

If the patient's lymphedema is due to breast cancer, consider mentioning the Women's Health and Cancer Rights Act (see WHCRA on page 71):

By limiting the number of lymphedema treatments, and thereby denying me medical coverage for complications due to breast cancer, <<*insurance plan*>> is violating federal law, specifically the Women's Health and Cancer Rights Act (WHCRA) P.L. 105-277 that was enacted on October 21, 1998.

Courtesy Copies

At the end there should be a list of others who are also receiving copies of this letter of appeal. This list should include the prescribing physician and others who may be able to influence the decision, the choice of insurance company, or the insurance company's business. For example:

- If insurance is provided by an employer, include the CEO or personnel director of the company.

- The Insurance Commissioner responsible for regulating insurance companies in your state.

- If you cite the WHCRA, include your senators and congressional representatives. See www.firstgov.gov for contact information.

It is important that these copies actually be sent. You may want to send a cover letter explaining the background and the reasons why you are sending them a copy of the letter.

Changing Insurance Plans

One of the most difficult situations to deal with in terms of health insurance is changing plans, for example if you take a new job, relocate, or if your spouse's coverage changes. When this need arises, there are factors that people with lymphedema should watch for. These include:

- Difficulty in finding insurance coverage.

- Restrictions on preexisting conditions for new members.

Finding Coverage

It may be difficult to find health insurance coverage if your situation changes. Consider all of your alternatives including:

- Continuing employee health benefits under COBRA or HIPAA, see page 68.

- Retirement benefits from the "good old days" of defined benefit plans that included health care coverage.

- Coverage through membership organizations like AARP or professional societies.

- Having your adult children list you as a dependent so you can be covered under their health insurance.

- Government benefits including Medicare or Medicaid. See www.GovBenefits.gov for information on federal and state benefits.

Preexisting Conditions

To the insurance company, a *preexisting condition* is an injury or illness that the patient had before changing to a new insurance plan. This is an important concept, because often the new plan will not cover expenses relating to a preexisting condition for as long as 12 months after the effective date of coverage. There are many variations of this clause and you need to look at the fine print of the policy to get the specifics. Some common examples are:

- A *preexisting condition* includes medical conditions known to the insured, even though no treatment was provided, during the designated period.

- A *preexisting condition* includes medical conditions that were diagnosed during a specified period, usually 3 or 6 months, before the new policy became effective.

- A *preexisting condition* includes medical conditions that required treatment during a specified period, usually 3 or 6 months, before the new policy became effective.

- A *preexisting condition* includes medical conditions that were diagnosed and required treatment during a specified period, usually 3 or 6 months, before the new policy became effective.

Legal Exceptions

If these laws apply, you may be able to avoid restrictions on preexisting conditions:

- You change from an employer plan to a self-paid plan via COBRA or HIPAA (see page 68).

- Your lymphedema is the result of breast cancer and you can apply the WHCRA (see page 71).

Care Without Coverage

If you are paying out of pocket for your care:

- Routine lymphedema treatment may be expensive, but the cost of treating complications, especially those requiring hospitalization, is much higher.

- Tell your health care providers if money is an issue. Enlist their help in prioritizing care, tests, and other medical expenses.

- Prices for medical care are not necessarily fixed. You may be able to negotiate a better price if you do so in advance and provide assurance of payment.

- You may be able to deduct these medical expenses on your income tax return, consult your tax advisor.

If you are unable to pay for care:

- Contact your local health department for information on indigent care.

- Research free medical clinics in your area. These may include charitable organizations, medical schools and other teaching institutions, etc.

Relevant Laws

Federal laws that may help people with lymphedema include:

- COBRA gives workers the right to continue group health coverage.

- HIPAA improves portability of health coverage.

- ADA requires businesses to accommodate people with disabilities.

- FMLA provides medical leave due to health conditions.

- WHCRA provides specific rights for breast cancer survivors.

Each of these laws is summarized below. Your state may also have helpful laws. Consult a lawyer or legal aid clinic for more information, this summary is not intended as legal advice.

COBRA

The Consolidated Omnibus Budget Reconciliation Act (COBRA) was passed by the US Congress in 1986.[1] This act gives workers who lose their jobs the right to continue group health benefits previously provided by their group health plan. This right continues only for a limited time period and the former employee must pay for this coverage.

COBRA Qualifying Events

COBRA provides certain former employees, retirees, spouses, former spouses, and dependent children the right to temporary continuation of health coverage at group rates when coverage is lost due to certain qualifying events.

Qualifying Events for Employees include: (1) voluntary or involuntary termination of employment for reasons other than gross misconduct; or (2) a reduction in the number of hours of employment.

Qualifying Events for Spouses include: (1) voluntary or involuntary termination of employment for reasons other than gross misconduct; (2) a reduction in the number of hours of employment; (3) covered employee becoming entitled to Medicare; (4) divorce or legal separation from the covered employee; or (5) death of the covered employee.

Qualifying Events for Dependent Children include: (1) loss of dependent child status under the plan rules; (2) voluntary or involuntary termination of the covered employee's employment for any reason other than gross misconduct; (3) reduction in the hours worked by the covered employee; (4) covered employee becoming entitled to Medicare; (5) divorce or legal separation of the covered employee; or (6) death of the covered employee.

COBRA Costs

Group health coverage for COBRA participants is usually more expensive than health coverage for active employees. This is because COBRA participants pay the entire premium but active employees typically have part of their premium paid by the employer. COBRA participants also pay a small administrative fee; however, the total cost for this coverage is ordinarily less than individual health coverage.

HIPAA

The federal Health Insurance Portability and Accountability Act (HIPAA) was signed into law in 1996 and offers protections for American workers by improving the portability and continuity of health insurance coverage.[2] It is especially useful for individuals who: (1) are at high risk, usually due to a pre-existing condition, (2) have had insurance through their jobs for at least 18 months, and (3) have exhausted their coverage under COBRA.

HIPAA includes protection for coverage under group health plans that limit exclusions for preexisting conditions, prohibit discrimination against employees and dependents based on their health status, and allow a special opportunity to enroll in a new plan to individuals in certain circumstances.

ADA

The Americans with Disabilities Act (ADA) is a federal law passed in 1990 that covers all businesses with 15 or more employees.[3] The purpose of this law is to protect individuals with disabilities. Under the law, disabled is defined as being someone who:

- Has a physical or mental impairment that substantially limits one or more major life activities.

- Has a record of such an impairment.

- Is regarded as having such an impairment.

Those with lymphedema who have limited mobility may be covered by this description. Under the terms of this law, *"the reasonable accommodations required by the Act include time off for medical treatment, flexible hours, and changes in duties to accommodate functional limitations."*

This accommodation must be requested on behalf of an employee with a disability by the employee, a family member, friend, health professional, rehabilitation counselor, or other representative. Although a written request is not required, it is prudent to put the request in writing and to keep a copy in your files.

FMLA

The Family and Medical Leave Act (FMLA) is a federal law passed in 1993 that covers all businesses that employ 50 or more people.[4] Although often thought of as providing unpaid leave following the birth or adoption of a child, coverage under this Act is much broader.

FMLA also provides up to 12 weeks of unpaid leave for workers *"to take medical leave when the employee is unable to work because of a serious health condition."* Under the terms of the law, this leave time does not have to be used all at once. Therefore a patient, such as someone with lymphedema who requires periodic treatment sessions, can take time off when as needed.

WHCRA

If lymphedema is the result of breast cancer, the patient has specific rights under the federal Women's Health and Cancer Rights Act (WHCRA) of 1998.[5] This law mandates that all insurance companies and HMOs provide coverage for *"physical complications of mastectomy including lymphedema."*

Note that WHCRA does not provide protection for patients covered by Medicare because Medicare is a government program, not insurance or an HMO.

Stories of Lymph Notes Members

- I need to find a treatment that works because my condition is worsening at an alarming rate. I walk only with great difficulty, yet my insurance company refuses coverage and I am in danger of being unable to work.

- I find it difficult to deal with my lymphedema physically and emotionally, but also in regards to insurance coverage and finding the answers that doctors don't have or take the time to study.

Chapter 6

Complications of Lymphedema

Lymphedema makes a person vulnerable to a variety of complications including:

- Infections of the skin and tissues including cellulitis, erysipelas, athlete's foot, and toenail fungus.

- Orthopedic problems caused by, or made worse by, lymphatic swelling.

- Tissue changes induced by lymphedema including fibrosis, hyperkeratosis, papillomatosis, and weeping lymphedema.

- Lymphangiosarcoma, a rare but deadly cancer of untreated lymphedema.

These complications can be painful, disabling, and even fatal. Treatment and self-management to minimize the swelling and promote overall health reduces the risk of all these complications.

Cellulitis and erysipelas are fast spreading infections that can quickly become life threatening medical emergencies. Patients with lymphedema, and those who care for them, must learn to recognize the symptoms of infection and know how to respond (see pages 75 and 77). Ongoing vigilance is an essential part of self-management and homecare.

Infections

In lymphedema the swelling of the affected limb or area is caused by stagnant protein-rich lymph—an ideal breeding ground for bacteria. Several types of bacteria that normally live on the surface of the skin can enter through the smallest break in the skin and cause potentially serious infections.

Swollen Glands or Lymph Nodes

The question most commonly asked by visitors to the Lymph Notes web site is, *"I have swollen glands. Does this mean that I have lymphedema?"* The answer to this question is, *"No, swollen glands are not a symptom of lymphedema."* However, it is also necessary to explain that swollen glands do occur in those with lymphedema (and others) when an infection is present.

One major role of the lymph nodes is to destroy any pathogens that the lymph has collected from the tissues. *Pathogens* are disease-producing microorganisms including bacteria, viruses, and cancer cells. A lymph node becomes swollen when specialized cells within the node have destroyed a large number of pathogens.

Swollen glands are more accurately described as *swollen lymph nodes* or by the medical term *lymphadenitis*. When someone with lymphedema develops swollen glands, it is necessary to look for other indications of an infection in the affected limb. If signs of infection are present, prompt medical treatment is required.

Cellulitis

Cellulitis, or *lymphangitis*, is a spreading bacterial infection of the skin and the tissues immediately beneath the skin.[1] This infection is caused by the bacteria *Staphylococcus* (commonly known as *staph)* or *Streptococcus* (commonly known as *strep*) that normally live harmlessly on the skin. However, even the smallest break in the skin may allow them to enter the body and cause an infection.

Because cellulitis spreads freely and uncontrollably through both the lymphatic and circulatory systems, and can spread to other body systems, it can quickly cause life-threatening damage. Cellulitis is more serious in individuals with underlying diseases such as diabetes, cancer, or immunodeficiency.

Cellulitis Symptoms

- A sudden increase in swelling

- Discoloration such as redness or streaky red lines in the skin

- Tissues that feel hot and tender

- Rash, itching

- Pain

- Chills and fever

- A feeling of general discomfort or uneasiness

- Achy flu-like symptoms

Cellulitis is a medical emergency that requires immediate treatment.

Cellulitis Treatment

Antibiotics are administered to control the infection and prevent complications. Most cellulitis infections are treated with oral antibiotics and outpatient follow-up. However, if the infection is severe or if other complications are present, hospitalization may be required for the intravenous administration of antibiotics and close observation to detect complications.

Penicillin-related antibiotics have traditionally been used for this purpose. However, treatment has become more difficult with the emergence of MRSA (*methicillin resistant staphylococcus aureus*), which is a strain of *Staphylococcus* that has developed resistance to penicillin-related antibiotics.[2]

These infections are so serious that some physicians prescribe antibiotics for their lymphedema patients to keep on hand at all times and instruct their patients to begin self-treatment immediately if they develop symptoms of an infection. If your doctor has given you this type of prescription:

☐ Do not wait for an infection to develop before you have the prescription filled.

☐ Be sure that you, and your caregivers, know when you should start taking these antibiotics and how much to take (the correct dosage).

☐ Seek medical care after beginning self-treatment. Contact your health-care provider or emergency services.

If you have any questions about this medication, check with your doctor.

Erysipelas

In contrast to cellulitis, which thrives within the deeper tissues, erysipelas attacks the tissues and lymphatic structures just under the surface of the skin. These painful infections most frequently occur on the lower legs (Figure 6.1).

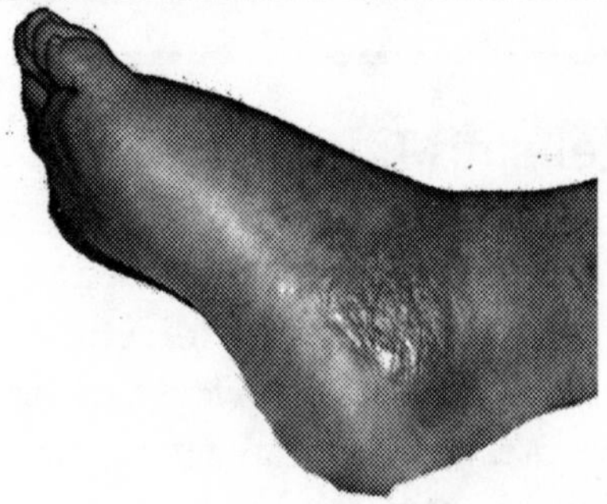

Erysipelas is usually caused by *Group A Streptococci*, which normally live harmlessly on the skin.[3] These bacteria invade rapidly through any break in the skin and spread through the lymphatic vessels.

This infection further disrupts the flow of lymph by damaging the lymphatic vessels and by increasing the fibrosis (hardening) within the infected tissues.

Figure 6-1: Erysipelas occurs most frequently on the lower leg.

Erysipelas Symptoms

- An expanding area of red skin that is warm and painful

- Chills and high fever

- Sores that typically have a raised border

- Blisters that develop over these sores

- Underlying skin that is intensely hardened and swollen

- Swelling and tenderness of the regional lymph nodes

Erysipelas Treatment

Erysipelas is also a serious infection that requires prompt medical treatment. Antibiotics, such as penicillin, that are effective against *Streptococci* are usually administered orally. If the infection is severe, intravenous antibiotics may be required. When individuals have recurrent erysipelas, long-term antibiotic treatment may be necessary as well.

Relieving the Itching of Erysipelas

If your health care provider approves, a cold wet pack can be used to relieve the itching associated with erysipelas. This cold pack consists of a clean cotton cloth, such as a towel, that is wet with cold water and wrapped around the inflamed limb. This lowers the temperature of the limb, eases the itching, and encourages healing.

Important: *Do not use an ice pack* for this purpose because it is too harsh against the tissues. Instead, use a clean cloth that is kept cold and moist by pouring more cold water over it.

Stories of Lymph Notes Members

Something else that has occurred is I got a couple of knots under my arm in the pit area and they got real red, swollen and hurt. I went to the Doc, he drained one and they called me today to tell me that he wants me to take a bunch of antibiotics because the swab came back with staph in it. Now I'm totally confused. I know that lymphedema causes the bacteria to stay in your arm until it's manually drained but could that be what caused the staph infection?

Athlete's Foot

Athlete's foot, which is an infection caused by the fungus *tinea pedis*, frequently occurs on the warm and moist tissues between the toes. As the infection spreads it may also be present on the soles or sides of the feet.[4]

For those with lymphedema of the legs and feet, athlete's foot is a major concern because it causes breaks in the skin. These cracks may allow bacteria to enter and cause erysipelas as a secondary infection.

Athlete's Foot Symptoms

- Red, dry, flaking skin

- Itching and pain

- Cracking of the skin between the toes

- Blistering

- Pustules (small raised areas containing pus)

- Weeping sores

Athlete's Foot Treatment

Although developing athlete's foot in a lymphedema-affected limb is not a medical emergency, it is necessary to seek medical care. The most commonly recommended treatment is a prescription-strength anti-fungal ointment.

Jock Itch

Jock itch is an infection caused by the fungus *tinea cruris*. Like athlete's foot, this fungus thrives in a warm moist environment. The difference is that jock itch occurs in the folds of the groin and in the creases between folds of skin as found in stage 3 lymphedema (see Figure 2-2). Jock itch is a serious hazard for those with lymphedema because it causes breakdown of the skin and creates openings where bacteria can enter and cause an infection.

Jock Itch Symptoms

- Rash that starts within the skin folds and progresses outward.

- Advancing edge of the infection is redder and more raised than areas that have been infected longer.

Jock Itch Treatment

Jock itch can be treated with over-the-counter ointments; however, it is advisable to see your physician for professional advice. Once the condition is under control, antifungal powders or sprays may be recommended for daily use as a preventive measure.

Toenail Fungus

A fungus infection of the toenail is another common problem for those with lower-extremity lymphedema. This condition, which is also known by the medical term *onychomycosis*, occurs because shoes and socks keep the toenails dark, warm, and moist—a perfect environment for fungus growth.

Toenail Fungus Symptoms

- Changes of the color of the nail to yellow-green or brown

- Flaking of the surface of the nail

- Debris collecting under the nail

- A bad smell coming from the nail

- Thickening of the nails

- Shoes that feel tight or short

- Pain when standing or walking

Toenail Fungus Treatment

A toenail fungus infection will not improve without treatment and professional foot care is strongly recommended.

Fish-Related Infections

Mycobacterium marinum is a slow growing bacterium that infects fish and people. This infection can be acquired by humans while cleaning fish tanks, swimming in ponds, lakes or streams, or handling fish.

Because *mycobacterium marinum* does not grow at normal body temperature, the infection remains localized near the cooler surface of the skin. The most frequent sign of an infection is a slowly developing nodule (raised bump) at the site where the bacteria entered the body. Later the nodule can enlarge and become an ulcer-like sore. As the disease progresses, nearby lymph nodes swell and multiple sores may form in a line along the lymphatic vessel that drains the site.

If your arm and hand are affected by lymphedema, the best approach is to have someone else clean the catch-of-the-day or the fish tank. If this isn't an option, wear long waterproof gloves that protect the hands and arms while performing these tasks. Also, avoid swimming in contaminated water.

Orthopedic Complications

Lymphedema may cause problems in muscles, tendons, and joints. Muscle strain can be caused by the added weight of the lymphedema and the associated loss of symmetry and changes in balance. Tendons that are flooded with lymphatic fluid can lose their elasticity and ability to glide smoothly, resulting in irritation and inflammation. Joints in the shoulder or pelvis may be destabilized by accumulated lymphatic fluid. In cases of secondary lymphedema, lymphatic swelling can make the underlying condition worse and complicate treatment.

Rotator cuff tendonitis is a complication of lymphedema caused by internal derangement of tendon fibers and may be treated effectively with anti-inflammatory drugs and physical therapy.[7] Frequent complications have been reported in post mastectomy patients undergoing surgical repair (*arthroplasty*) of the shoulder, especially those with pre-operative lymphedema.[8]

Tissue Changes

If lymphedema progresses from Stage 1 through Stage 3, serious changes occur within the tissues and on the skin. These changes can be treated; however, they cannot always be completely reversed.

Stories of Lymph Notes Members

I was diagnosed with lymphedema 12 years ago. I am only 43 and have been dragging this heavy leg, and sometimes both legs, to work. I bandage, exercise, and watch my diet. About once a year I participate in a six week daily massage at the lymphedema clinic in the city.

Until now: now I have injured my back from constantly being twisted and strained because of my leg. I have now dislocated my left leg from the hip, dislocated my pelvic bone, and have three herniated discs.

Fibrosis

Fibrosis is abnormal hardening of the deeper tissues below the skin. Tissues that have hardened in this manner are referred to as being *fibrotic*.

In lymphedema, fibrosis occurs as an inflammatory reaction to the presence of stagnant, protein-rich lymph. Fibrosis of the skin can also be caused by radiation, burns, or chronic wounds. The changes of fibrosis further slow the lymph circulation within the affected area; this traps more stagnant lymph and causes additional swelling. As this process progresses, skin changes occur that increase the risk of infection. Some fibrosis can be reversed with treatment but the longer the condition has been present, the less effective treatment tends to be.

Skin Changes

Uncontrolled lymphedema steadily compromises the health of the skin by reducing its flexibility and changing its texture.[5] Some of the skin changes associated with lymphedema are hyperkeratosis, papillomatosis, and weeping lymphedema.

Hyperkeratosis

Hyperkeratosis is abnormal thickening of the outer layer of the skin that causes the skin to lose its elasticity. This, combined with ever-increasing lymphatic swelling, causes the skin to hang in folds (see Figure 2.2).

Papillomatosis

Papillomatosis is a condition in which hard, noncancerous growths form on the surface of the skin. These growths, which are close together, give the skin a rough appearance like the bark of a tree, and may cause abnormal flaking of the outer layer of the skin.[6]

Weeping Lymphedema

Weeping lymphedema occurs most often in Stage 3 lymphedema, particularly in affected legs. Also known as *lymphorrhea*, this condition is characterized by the flow of lymph through the skin. This flow can be rapid enough to run or trickle down the leg, where the lymph further irritates the skin and increases the patient's risk of developing cellulitis.

Open Wounds and Cracks in the Skin

Open wounds can develop within the warm, moist skin folds that are common in Stage 3 lymphedema. This skin is not healthy and fungal infections can cause openings in the skin. These openings permit bacteria to enter and cause infections.

Lymphangiosarcoma

Lymphangiosarcoma is a rare, but usually fatal, complication of long-standing, untreated primary or secondary lymphedema. This cancer originates in the lymphedema affected area and spreads rapidly to other parts of the body.

Stories of Lymph Notes Members

- I was treated for ovarian cancer in 1979. The lymphedema began in 1980 and it escalated in 1991. My left leg is probably 150 pounds of fluid and the right leg is now increasing. The left leg is so swollen that I have leakage of lymph in two areas.

- I was treated for melanoma in 1974. In 1976 I developed lymphedema in my right leg. I had a successful pregnancy in 1990. In 1994 an insect bite made my leg much worse and I started treatment that year. Since then, at one time or another, I have used MLD, a pump, ReidSleeve, Circ-Aid, various garments, Coumarin and Venalot (from Germany). I'm always looking for fashionable shoes for my mismatched feet. I'm also interested in finding constructive strategies for dealing with the issues around lymphedema.

Chapter **7**

Lymphedema and Other Conditions

Some medical conditions cause secondary lymphedema to develop as a complication. Understanding common disorders that can cause secondary lymphedema and the interactions of both conditions is important because it impacts the treatment and potential outcome.[1]

People with lymphedema run the usual risks of developing other health issues. Although lymphedema may not cause this disorder, the presence of both disorders at the same time can require modification of the lymphedema treatment.

Obesity

Obesity is an excess of fat in proportion to lean body mass results in weight that is generally considered to be unhealthy for a given height. Although lymphatic fluid is dense and swelling will cause weight gain, not everyone with lymphedema becomes obese. However, lymphedema can lead to obesity when a person gains weight due to the lack of exercise, the loss of mobility, or unhealthy eating patterns associated with depression.

Conversely, not everyone with obesity develops lymphedema. However, lymphedema can develop as a complication of obesity. Obesity is associated with a variety of health problems as discussed in Chapter 14.

Living Well With Lymphedema   **85**

The Treatment of Obesity and Lymphedema

A patient with obesity-related conditions, including lymphedema, presents a complex diagnostic challenge. The medical problems must be identified and prioritized so that the most serious conditions can be treated first. It is only after the more serious conditions are under control that lymphedema treatment can be safely performed.

Is the Patient Ready for Treatment?

Another issue that needs to be addressed with the obese patient is, *"Are you ready, willing, and able to be an active participant in your lymphedema treatment?"* Patient cooperation is essential to a good outcome. A patient who is willing and able to perform the lymphedema self-management tasks has a much better chance of achieving improvement in both conditions.

Treatment Modifications

When an obese patient is treated for lymphedema, it is frequently necessary to modify the usual Complete Decongestive Therapy program.

- **Bandaging and the use of other compression aids** are contraindicated for some obese patients because the amount of fluid returned to the cardiovascular system creates too much strain on the heart. When the patient's heart is able to tolerate some additional load, bandaging may be helpful when it is modified to extend only to the knee instead of bandaging up to the hip.

- **Exercise,** as tolerated, is essential to stimulate the flow of lymph and as part of a weight reduction program.

Lipedema

Lipedema, also known as *painful fat syndrome*, is an inherited disorder that affects mostly women and is characterized by abnormal fatty deposits lo-

Stories of Lymph Notes Members

I am 56 and my legs have been huge for years. I was told on my second day post-op from gastric bypass surgery that I have lymphedema.

cated below the skin of the hips and legs, down to the ankles.

Lymphedema does not cause lipedema. Lipedema can cause lymphedema as a complication of the later stages.

The Diagnosis of Lipedema

Lipedema is often confused with obesity or lymphedema, particularly in the later stages, and this makes an accurate diagnosis of lipedema more difficult. The symptoms of lipedema include:

- In the early stages of lipedema, the upper part of the body may be slim. Despite a slender upper body, fat accumulates from the tops of the hips to the ankles; the feet are not involved.[2]

- When weight is gained, it accumulates in the lipedema affected areas of the hips and legs.

- When weight is lost, the fat decrease occurs in areas other than those affected by lipedema. The weight is not lost from the area between the waist and the ankles.

- Fat extends down the legs and creates a ring of fatty tissue that may overlap the tops of the feet.

- Swelling in the legs develops during the second half of the day. This swelling decreases during sleep.

- Pain is present, particularly along the shin.

- *Nodules,* which are small fatty lumps within the tissues, develop in the early stages.

- *Lobules,* which are rounded fat deposits, larger than nodules and near the surface of the skin, develop in the later stages.

Characteristics that distinguish lipedema from lymphedema include:

- Lipedema tends to be more symmetric than lymphedema.

- Lipedema patients often complain of pain when touched.

- Lipedema is prone to bruising and subcutaneous bleeding which is absent in lymphedema.

- Lipedema is not prone to the infections typical of lymphedema.

- The absence of a Stemmer's Sign and swelling in the foot.

Complications of Lipedema

- **Obesity** is the most common complication of lipedema; approximately half of all lipedema patients are obese.[3] As more weight is gained, additional stresses are placed on all body systems.

- **Secondary lymphedema** affecting the legs is a complication as lipedema progresses in the later stages. A positive Stemmer's sign (see page 22) may indicate the presence of lymphedema.

- **Lipo-lymphedema** is the combination of lipedema, obesity, and lymphedema. Lipo-lymphedema can also develop in combination with idiopathic edema, chronic venous insufficiency, and other vascular diseases. *Idiopathic edema* is swelling of unknown cause.

The Treatment of Lipedema and Lymphedema

When lipedema and lymphedema are present concurrently, the lymphedema therapist must balance the needs of both conditions.

- **Manual lymph drainage** is used initially with only very light strokes because of the pain associated with lipedema. These gentle strokes open the superficial lymphatics (located just under the skin) and decrease the pain by clearing blocked draining areas and clogged lymph nodes. After several sessions, when the pain is less, the therapist can start working on the affected limbs.

- **Bandaging and compression garments** are not applied until the patient is able to tolerate compression without pain.

Congestive Heart Failure

Congestive heart failure (CHF), which occurs most often in the elderly, is a condition in which the heart is unable to pump out all of the blood that it receives. This decreased pumping action of the heart causes congestion[4] (fluid buildup):

- **Left-sided heart failure**, also known as pulmonary edema, causes fluid buildup in the lungs.

- **Right-sided heart failure** causes fluid buildup beginning with the feet and legs. This swelling can also affect the liver, gastrointestinal tract, or arms.

Congestive heart failure is treated with medications to control blood pressure, to strengthen the heart beat, and to reduce the fluid load. Patients may be advised to keep their legs elevated or to wear compression stockings to minimize swelling. This reduces the pressure on the heart and veins and allows fluid to return to the cardiovascular system.

Lymphedema is not linked to congestive heart failure in the medical literature.

Congestive Heart Failure and Lymphedema

The swelling due to right-sided congestive heart failure causes fluid retention in the tissues of the feet and legs. This excess fluid must be transported by the lymphatic system and this added stress can cause a CHF patient to develop secondary lymphedema of the lower extremities as a complication.

Just as with others in the general population, an individual with lymphedema can develop congestive heart failure. If CHF develops, it is diagnosed and treated by the patient's physician. As with any change in medical condition, the patient's lymphedema therapist should be informed promptly.

Treatment of Congestive Heart Failure and Lymphedema

When both conditions are present, the patient's health care provider must be consulted before lymphedema treatment starts.

- **Manual lymph drainage** may be contraindicated if it places too much strain on the heart by increasing the volume of circulating blood.

- **Bandaging** may be contraindicated, or must be modified, because it too increases the strain on the heart.

- **Compression stockings** are used in the treatment of congestive heart failure; however, these stockings *are not* the same compression strength as the stockings used in the treatment of lymphedema.

- **Exercise**, as tolerated by the patient, is recommended to improve heart function, venous circulation, and lymphatic drainage.

Chronic Venous Insufficiency

Chronic venous insufficiency (CVI) is a condition in which the veins of the legs do not efficiently return blood to the heart. This may be due to improper functioning of the valves in the veins, the blockage of one or more veins in the lower legs, or a combination of these conditions.

CVI results in pooling of blood in the legs and feet, and causes symptoms that include dull aching pain and a feeling of heaviness or cramping. Swelling of the legs with low-protein fluid is also present. This swelling occurs in the second half of the day and is known as *dependent edema* or *orthostatic edema*. Swelling is often the result of standing for long periods of time; this type of swelling usually goes away overnight or with exercise.

Lymphedema does not cause chronic venous insufficiency.

CVI and Lymphedema

The slowed circulation and swelling of chronic venous insufficiency places added stress on the lymphatic system in the lower extremities. These stresses may cause secondary lymphedema to develop as a complication of CVI.

Like others in the general population, an individual with lymphedema can develop chronic venous insufficiency due to causes that are not associated with lymphedema.

Treatment of CVI and Lymphedema

- Manual lymph drainage brings relief to the venous system and improves the functioning of the lymphatic system.

- Compression is used to control the swelling of chronic venous insufficiency. If bandaging is required, short-stretch bandages are used for patients who are able to walk and exercise. As explained in Chapter 4, long-stretch bandages are used for patients who are unable to walk.

Diabetes

Diabetes is a chronic condition in which the body does not produce, or use, insulin properly. Diabetes is characterized by uncontrolled blood sugar levels and can be a life-threatening disorder until the blood sugar levels are controlled.[5]

The causes of diabetes are not clearly understood but they appear to include heredity and obesity. Lymphedema does not cause diabetes. Like others in the general population, an individual with lymphedema may also develop diabetes due to factors that are unrelated to lymphedema.

Poorly controlled diabetes affects the cardiovascular system, resulting in reduced oxygen levels in the skin, the underlying subcutaneous tissues, and the deeper connective tissues. This makes these tissues extremely fragile and prone to open sores. When lymphedema is also present, it further damages these tissues and increases the risk of infections such as cellulitis.

Diabetes and Lymphedema Treatment

When an individual with lymphedema also has diabetes, treatment must be modified to accommodate the conditions caused by the diabetes:

- **Manual lymph drainage and self-massage** are performed with great care to protect the very thin, fragile, and dry skin associated with diabetes.

- **Before bandaging**, the therapist, or patient, should carefully examine the tissues to be bandaged for any signs of circulatory problems. Self-bandaging is not performed if there are indications of circulatory difficulties. The therapist uses his or her professional judgment about proceeding with this treatment.

- **Bandaging and the use of compression garments** are modified to avoid skin irritation. Ointment or powder may be used to relieve the itching associated with the dry skin related to diabetes.

- **Excellent skin care** including moisturizing the skin with a lotion—such as Eucerin® Original—before bandaging will help minimizing itching and reduce the risk of infection. Skin Care is discussed in Chapter 9.

Testing Blood Glucose Levels

Glucose monitoring requires a blood sample that is obtained by using a tiny lancet to prick the skin of the finger or forearm. Testing should not be done on tissues affected by lymphedema or at risk for it.

The sides of the fingers are frequently used for blood glucose testing. When the arm is affected by lymphedema or is at risk for it, these sites are not a safe choice. For example, 30 years after a mastectomy, a newly diagnosed diabetic began performing finger stick tests on the fingers of her "at risk" arm. Within a matter of days she had developed lymphedema in that arm.[6]

Insulin Injections

Some diabetics inject insulin into the layer of fat located just under the skin of the abdomen, thighs, hip, or buttocks. Since injections should not be made into lymphedema-affected tissues, a diabetic should ask his or her physician to recommend safe injection sites.

Peripheral Neuropathy

Peripheral neuropathy is damage to the nerves of the extremities (arms and hands or feet and legs). Nerve damage can be caused by diseases such as diabetes, as a side-effect of chemotherapy, or as the result of an injury.

The symptoms of peripheral neuropathy are usually experienced first as tingling and numbness in the hands or feet. As the damage progresses the sensations are described as burning, throbbing, aching, and "feels like frost-bite" or "walking on a bed of coals."

Peripheral Neuropathy and Lymphedema

Lymphedema does not cause peripheral neuropathy. Cancer patients that have had chemotherapy can develop both peripheral neuropathy and lymph-edema as secondary conditions. When both conditions are present, it is necessary to modify the lymphedema treatment to accommodate the patient's pain and inability to feel abnormal pressure against the tissues:

- Bandages and compression garments must be placed with great care to prevent rubbing or excessive pressure.

- The skin must be examined frequently to detect any signs of injury or infection.

Tingling and Burning Sensations of Lymphedema

Unpleasant sensations similar to the tingling and burning of peripheral neuropathy can occur in areas affected by lymphedema, even when peripheral neuropathy is not present. These sensations can be due to any number of causes including improper compression garment fit, swelling, fibrosis, and problems elsewhere in the body as explained below.

Improper Fitting of Compression Garment

A compression garment that does not fit properly can cause these symptoms. If you suspect this is the problem, try removing the garment and replacing it with bandages. Bandages have the advantage that they can be adjusted to your comfort level. Therefore, they should not cause numbness, tingling, or pain.

If the problem seems to be related to your compression garment, have your therapist check the fit of this garment. A new compression garment may be necessary.

Swelling and Fibrosis

The swelling of lymphedema, and the hardened tissues of fibrosis, can put pressure on nerves in the affected area. If you have these symptoms, mention them to your therapist to determine if changes in your treatment regimen might help.

Problems Located Elsewhere in Your Body

It is possible that problems located elsewhere in your body could be causing the unpleasant sensations in the lymphedema-affected area. Neck problems, muscle spasms, overuse injuries, and a host of other causes can create these tingling sensations and feelings of discomfort. If these sensations are causing serious discomfort, and lymphedema related causes have been ruled out, it is necessary to have potential causes investigated.

As part of the diagnostic process, an electromyograph test may be recommended. *Electromyography* is used to evaluate the electrical activity in a muscle. This test requires placing very thin needles into the muscle fibers. Because these needles go through the skin it is advisable to avoid having this test performed on lymphedema-affected tissues.

Reminder

- Some of these conditions can cause secondary lymphedema. The risks of this happening depends on your overall health, age, and heredity.

- Having lymphedema does not necessarily increase the likelihood of your developing other conditions.

- Lymphedema treatment and self-management will improve your overall health and minimize your risk of developing additional conditions.

Chapter **8**

The Emotional Challenges of Lymphedema

Lymphedema brings emotional as well as physical challenges.[1] Your response to these emotional challenges affects your quality of life in many ways. How you handle these emotions impacts your actions and your enjoyment of life. It affects your willingness to initiate and maintain your self-management plan, day after day. It influences your relationships and how you feel about yourself.

I want to give you a "road map" for charting the emotional terrain of having lymphedema. Like any useful map, it will let you know what to expect, give you directions about how to navigate to reach your destination, and provide warning signs of dangerous areas and indicators that you may have gotten off the track.

This chapter will:

- Summarize the most common emotional reactions to lymphedema,

- Provide coping tips, and

- Explain the warning signs of problematic emotional reactions.

> **Publisher's Note:** Dr. McMahon's book, **Overcoming the Emotional Challenges of Lymphedema,** addresses this topic in more depth, covers a wider range of emotional challenges, provides more detail about coping tips, and teaches more advanced skills; as well as providing information for friends and family, psychotherapists, and medical professionals.

Predictable Emotional Reactions

Does any of this sound familiar to you?

- ☐ I'm angry! I hate having lymphedema! I hate the problem and the people who caused it! I hate that the doctors didn't warn me about it and can't fix it.

- ☐ Lymphedema has taken things away from me. I can't do things I used to enjoy. I feel so sad I want to cry.

- ☐ I'm scared! What's safe and what's not? Will something else go wrong next?

- ☐ My clothes don't fit. I don't like these changes in my body. I am self-conscious. I feel uncomfortable being sexual. What am I supposed to tell people?

- ☐ Why did this happen to me? It's not fair. I can't believe this happened.

- ☐ Sometimes I feel overwhelmed! I can't do this. I want to give up. It's too much.

If these thoughts and feelings sound familiar, take heart. You are not alone. These are normal reactions.

Lymphedema Isn't Just Physical

Having lymphedema means that you have a chronic condition. You didn't choose it. You don't like it. And there's no going back.

At times, you may feel scared, confused, sad, or angry. You may feel trapped, helpless, and betrayed. These are all normal reactions to having a chronic condition.

The bad news is that these reactions, although normal and predictable, are painful and distressing. The good news is that you can cope with them. The more you know about what to expect, the less you will be blindsided by your emotions. The more skillfully you cope with them, the less of a problem they will present over time.

It All Fits Together

Our emotions and thoughts, our actions and our body, all affect each other both directly and indirectly. Change one and you affect the other:

- How skillfully you cope with natural reactions influences how disruptive they are and how intensely they impact your emotional state.

- Your emotional state affects how well you care for your lymphedema. In turn, how you care for yourself affects both the state of your lymphedema and your emotional well-being.

- The state of your lymphedema affects you physically and emotionally. In their turn, these factors influence your level of activity.

- Your level of activity impacts both your lymphedema and your emotions.

In other words, in order to live well with lymphedema you need to cope with your emotions and your physical symptoms.

What's Normal? What's Not?

To some degree, the specific emotional challenges created by lymphedema vary from person to person. At the same time, certain reactions occur often enough to be considered normal and predictable.

Normal Emotional Reactions

These challenging emotional reactions frequently occur with lymphedema:

- Anger

- Sadness and grief

- Struggling to make sense of what has happened

- Anxiety and worry

- Self-consciousness

- Feeling overwhelmed

Everyone who has faced lymphedema has struggled with at least some of these reactions. Remember, others have been through this and have dealt successfully with these emotions. You have companions on this journey. You don't have to be a helpless victim of these natural reactions.

Problematic Emotional Reactions

The normal emotional reactions above are distressing. Distressing feelings are never pleasant or welcomed, but they are not necessarily problematic.

Unpleasant emotions are actually designed to be helpful. They alert us to problems. They motivate us to make changes. They help us monitor our progress. Distressing emotions should subside as we face our challenges successfully.

Sometimes, however, emotions are so intense, prolonged, or one-sided that they stop being helpful. Instead, the emotions themselves, or our responses to them, create problems. Look for these warning signs that your emotions may have become problematic.

Warning Signs

Be concerned if your emotions are:

☐ Getting worse, not better, with time

☐ Harming your quality of life

☐ Interfering with your self-management

☐ Disrupting your relationships with family and friends

☐ Interfering with your general functioning

☐ Causing you to do things that are harmful or dangerous

If you are experiencing problematic emotional reactions, talk to a mental health professional. Also consider talking to a professional if you feel that your emotional reactions are normal, but they are not improving as the months pass.

The rest of this chapter addresses the normal emotional challenges, one at a time. It reviews what you can expect, gives tips on coping, and covers the emotion-specific warning signs.

Anger

Anger or resentment is often one of the first responses, and it can be one of the longest lasting. It is normal to react to being diagnosed with lymphedema by having such thoughts as: "Why me?" "Why are other people healthy and

I'm not?" "Why didn't my doctor warn me, prevent this, or diagnose it earlier?" "Why isn't there a cure?" "I hate this!" "It isn't fair." "I hate this thing and the people who caused it!"

Anger is useful when you face a physical fight; it stirs you up physically and prepares you to attack. It is natural, but not very helpful, when you face a chronic disease. How can you cope with it?

Coping with Anger

To cope with anger, you must understand what is causing it. Anger is what is called a "secondary emotion." In other words, *we get angry in response to some other underlying emotion, usually fear or hurt.*

Discover the real problem:

- Ask yourself, "What do I fear will happen? Why am I feeling hurt?"

- Write out, or talk out, your anger in a safe way.

- Step back and ask yourself, "What are the real issues?"

Once you have uncovered the real underlying issues or emotions that triggered your anger, deal with them:

- You may be confronting a loss and defending against the pain and sorrow by getting angry.

- You may need to come to terms with something that is out of your control and that frightens you or makes you feel threatened or diminished.

- If you are angry about a situation, you may need to problem-solve or change your actions.

- If you are angry with another person, you may need to talk with that person. Emphasize the feelings and concerns underneath your anger.

Problem-solve with them. If possible, talk with the person as if he or she were a teammate, not an enemy.

Anger: Warning Signs

Pay attention to these warning signs that anger has become problematic:

- You are being destructive or acting in ways that are dangerous. Anger is being channeled into destruction instead of being harnessed for problem solving.

- You are being verbally abusive, screaming at others, name-calling, or threatening to hurt people.

- You are being physically abusive, shoving, pushing, slapping, punching, hitting, or choking others or threatening them with weapons. Treat this as an emergency and seek help immediately.

Psychotherapy or anger management training, possibly combined with medication, can help. Ideally, you should seek help from a professional who is trained and experienced in working with anger problems.

Sadness and Grief

It is very natural to feel sorrow and to grieve when you are diagnosed with lymphedema. Lymphedema brings unwanted life changes.

You now need to care actively for your body. You have to think more about what you do and how you do it. You have to take responsibility for a part of your body's functioning that used to work automatically. You have lost the luxury of taking part in many physical activities without thinking.

You may cry or feel numb. You may withdraw from people or reach out to them more. You may find it difficult to put lymphedema aside and enjoy yourself.

Overcoming Sadness and Grief

Permit yourself to grieve your losses. Let yourself cry.

Talk to people who understand and accept and who make you feel better. Avoid talking to people who make you feel worse.

Practice relaxation, deep breathing, and exercise. Exercise lifts your mood at the same time that it helps your lymphedema.

Actively seek out pleasure. You can do this in several ways:

- Fill your day with small pleasures. Really enjoy your cup of tea or coffee. Deliberately notice beauty around you. Actively savor little pleasures of life that are normally ignored. Our level of happiness is influenced by the small things in our lives, not just the big things.

- Wherever possible, regain lost pleasures. Write down any activities you used to enjoy that you no longer do because of lymphedema. Look for ways to bring these activities back into your life. Can you do them if you wear gloves, if you modify the intensity or duration of the activity, or if you take other protective actions?

- When that is not possible, replace lost pleasures with new ones. See Chapter 16 for ideas.

- Find meaningful activities and participate in them. Do things that give you a sense of accomplishment.

Sadness and Grief: Warning Signs

Natural sadness and grief are part of the process of adapting and adjusting to unwanted life changes. You grieve losses in order to come to terms with them so that you can move forward and rebuild a satisfying life—one that brings you joy and is of value. Sadness and grief lessen as you make appropriate changes and rediscover, or create, sources of pleasure and satisfaction.

However, normal sadness and grief can become problematic and turn into depression. Depression is when feelings of sorrow and grief are prolonged over time and interfere with your happiness and/or your functioning.

Depression is common with lymphedema and can be a serious problem. Depression can undermine your emotional health and your self-management by sapping your energy, disrupting your sleep, and making you feel hopeless. Depression can even be life threatening if it makes you so unhappy and hopeless that you feel suicidal.

Here are some warning signs of depression:

- You find yourself wanting to die.

- You feel worthless, guilty, or hopeless.

- You don't find pleasure in things you used to enjoy.

- You are either so agitated or so slowed down that others see the difference in you.

- You have trouble concentrating. You have less energy. Your sleep and/or appetite have increased or decreased.

If you have any of these warning signs, seek help.

The good news about depression is that effective treatments are available. Treatment may involve specific psychotherapies for depression (often cognitive-behavioral or interpersonal therapy), anti-depressant medication, or both. Talk to a mental health professional. Thousands of people with depression have gotten better.

Struggling to Make Sense of What Has Happened

When something bad happens to us, we try to make sense out of it. We struggle with natural questions like, "Why did this happen to me?" "Did I contribute to this?" "Did others contribute to this?" "How can I reconcile this with my philosophy of life, my religious beliefs, or my sense of justice?" "How does this affect my beliefs about the world, about other people, and about myself and my future?"

Making Sense of What Has Happened

To make sense of what has happened, it helps if you explore your thoughts and feelings. Don't just recite the facts of what has happened.

You can explore by talking with others who are nonjudgmental and helpful or through writing.

The key principle in writing is that it should feel safe to put your thoughts and feelings down on paper. You need to feel free to explore anything, knowing that what you write will not be used to hurt you or anyone else. If you keep a journal of health information to share with your doctors, you want to keep this writing some place else.

Some people like to keep a personal journal of feelings and insights and to review their writings over time. They find a safe place to store this journal.

Other people prefer to write and then immediately destroy what they have written. They feel freer and safer writing this way.

As you talk or write, try to place what has happened in a larger context. Adjust or enlarge your view of yourself, your view of the world, and your religious belief or philosophy of life to take lymphedema into account.

Deliberately turn your attention to finding ways to live the best life that you can under these new circumstances. You can't change the past. You can change the future by changing what you do now. This is your challenge.

Books such as *Writing Out The Storm*[2] by Barbara Abercrombie or *Opening Up*[3] by James Pennebaker, PhD can be helpful.

Making Sense of What Has Happened: Warning Signs

Here are warning signs that your attempts to meet this emotional challenge have become derailed and are causing problems:

- You can't get over what has happened. You keep reliving what happened, stay constantly tense, or feel cut off from normal feelings.

- You take all of the blame on yourself. You focus on your guilt and believe that you deserve to suffer.

- You decide that all other people are evil. You trust no one.

- You are unable to fit the existence of this illness and tragedy into your view of the world.

If you recognize these warning signs, seek help. You may consider attending a support group, seeing a spiritual counselor, and/or speaking with a licensed psychotherapist, especially one who has training and experience working with people who have faced medical illness or traumas.

Anxiety and Worry

It is natural to be scared and to worry about what might go wrong next. In fact, it is healthy to have a realistic level of anxiety and worry. Such feelings motivate you to get treatment, do self-management, and change your activities to protect yourself.

You face questions such as, "What's safe for me to do and what's dangerous?" "What is a sign of a problem?" "What can I safely ignore?" "What do I need to do for my health?" "What does that cut, bump, fever, or sensation mean?"

Managing Anxiety and Worry

Start by identifying all of your fears and worries. Write them all down even if you know they are unlikely.

Next, seek out and write down all the information and facts you can find that are relevant to your fears. For example, see Chapter 6 to learn the signs of lymphedema emergencies and what to do.

Using the information you have collected, critically evaluate how likely your fears really are. Compare what your fears say to what the facts say.

Identify other problems that could be troubling you. Sometimes anxiety occurs because we have issues in our lives that we are not addressing.

Occasionally, anxiety is a side effect of a medication or a medical condition. If you think this is the case, ask your healthcare team.

Think about the problem that's causing you anxiety. Look at it from all angles. Ask yourself these questions:

- What are the facts?

- What would someone who loved and accepted me advise me to do?

- What advice would I give someone in a similar situation?

Take every action to solve the real problems you face. When you identify a health risk, problem-solve ways to avoid it or reduce its damaging effects on your body.

Change what is under your control. Face and accept what is out of your control. There are some things—and people—that we just can't change.

Accept that you have to live with some uncertainty. We all have to tolerate uncertainty in our lives.

If worry still continues to trouble you throughout the day:

- Schedule a daily 'worry time' for about 20-30 minutes during which you do your whole day's worth of worrying.

- When worries pop up at other times, note them, ask them to wait, and then focus on them in your next worry time.

Anxiety and Worry: Warning Signs

Living well with lymphedema is a balancing act. On the one hand, you must stay realistically alert for problems and think about how to maintain and protect your body's health. On the other hand, you want to be able to relax and enjoy life.

Here are some signs that anxiety and worry have gotten out of balance:

- You worry constantly, even when the facts are reassuring.

- You worry about things that other people with lymphedema don't worry about.

- Your fears interfere with everyday functioning or keep you from following the advice of your healthcare professionals.

- You have panic attacks and worry about having more. Fear of panic attacks keeps you from doing things.

If you recognize these warning signs, consult a mental health professional who has training and experience treating anxiety.

There are very effective treatments for anxiety. In particular, cognitive-behavioral psychotherapy has been proven to be effective for anxiety and medication may also help some people with anxiety.

Self-Consciousness

Lymphedema changes your relationship with your body and your view of yourself. You may dress differently. You may act differently with others. You may even avoid being with others. You may have trouble feeling attractive or sexual.

You may wonder what other people think and how they will react. What will you say to them? Family and friends may not understand. They may not offer the help you want. Your boss or coworkers may wonder if you can do your job. Strangers may stare or ask questions. How can you deal with these challenges and feel good about yourself?

Managing Self-Consciousness

First of all, remember that you are more than your physical body. *You are more than your lymphedema.*

Remind yourself of all the things that make you a unique and worthwhile human being:

- List your skills, your accomplishments, and your talents.

- List your good qualities.

- Talk to yourself the way someone would if they knew you completely and loved and accepted you unconditionally.

- Live up to that view of yourself.

The Problems With Avoidance

Self-consciousness may make you want to avoid difficult—but important—interactions or conversations with others. For example, you may avoid discussing lymphedema. You may avoid asking for help from your family or others. You may even be tempted to avoid other people entirely.

Avoidance is a bad strategy for several reasons:

- It prevents you from learning that other people's reactions can be positive.

- It prevents you from learning and practicing ways to handle other people's reactions, no matter what they are.

- It keeps you self-conscious.

- It limits your life.

- It harms your view of yourself and your self-esteem.

Lymphedema is only one part of you. Don't let it control how you deal with other people.

Basic Communication Skills

Here are four basic communication skills for important or difficult conversations.[4] If the other person is a stranger, you may choose to use skill #2 only. For other conversations, you will probably wish to use all four.

1. Listen respectfully to the other person. Accept how they feel and what they want, especially when their feelings or goals are different from yours. Check that you have heard them correctly, even if you completely disagree, by summarizing what they think and feel.

2. Say how you feel and what you want in a way that is as easy as possible for them to understand. Stand your ground. Respect and accept your feelings as much as theirs.

3. Look for anything in what they say that you can honestly agree with and tell them that you agree with it. Honestly admit any way in which you contribute to the problem.

4. Problem-solve as a team. Find solutions that are at least minimally acceptable to everyone involved.

Now let's turn to specific issues that often arise in dealing with others. Here are some tips when dealing with family members or friends, dealing with sexual partners, dealing with acquaintances, bosses, or strangers, and dealing with caregivers or healthcare professionals.

Dealing with Family Members or Friends

Express your concerns and feelings to those who are close to you. Listen to their thoughts and feelings in return. Ask your family and friends for what you want. If they can't give it to you, take responsibility and get what you need somewhere else.

Be prepared to explain. Be patient. It may help to have someone else explain lymphedema and tell them what they can do to help you. They may find reading this book helpful.

Just like you, your family can feel impatient or 'burned out' by dealing with lymphedema. Try to understand and talk things out so that you face these problems together instead of having lymphedema divide you.

Family members who have successfully coped with chronic illness report that their relationship has grown deeper and that their happiness has increased. Working through emotional and practical problems can lead to greater respect, confidence, and trust.

Dealing with Sexual Partners

If you have trouble being sexual, discuss your concerns with your partner. Deliberately focus on thoughts that increase your arousal. Pay attention to experiencing whatever pleasure occurs in the moment without comparing it to the past or worrying about the future.

Try different positions. Experiment and find what works for you both. Give yourselves time because part of the body's response to physical stress is less interest in sexual activity.

Dealing with Acquaintances, Bosses, or Strangers

For acquaintances, bosses, and strangers, decide in advance what you want to tell them about your lymphedema. Practice your answers until you can say them comfortably and firmly in a pleasant tone. Practice smiling and maintaining eye contact.

Dealing with Caregivers or Healthcare Professionals

Use the basic communication skills and take responsibility for taking care of your health:

- Prepare. Write down your questions (see Chapter 15). Bring a copy for the other person. Educate yourself and get accurate information.

- Prioritize. Decide what is most important to you.

- Speak up. Only you know your needs and your questions.

- Listen. Understand their point of view even when you disagree. Ask them to repeat or clarify if you can't hear or understand them.

- Problem-solve together.

Self-Consciousness: Warning Signs

Some increased self-consciousness and change in self-image is predictable. Here are some warning signs that this issue has become problematic:

- You fear possible reactions from others or you don't know what to say.

- Self-consciousness stops you from asking others for what you need.

- You avoid others because you don't want them to see that you have lymphedema.

- You feel worthless or ugly.

- You desire the closeness of sexual intimacy, but feel that you have no choice but to avoid it out of self-consciousness or shame.

Problems with self-consciousness, with self-image, or with other people can stem from many different sources. If you notice these warning signs, consider seeking help from a mental health professional.

Feeling Overwhelmed

You have been diagnosed with a condition that many people have never heard of before. There is currently no cure and your lymphedema will get worse if you don't care for it. Suddenly you feel and look different. You have to learn new information. You have to change how you carry out your daily activities. You have to begin daily self-management.

No wonder there are times when you feel overwhelmed and think, "I can't do this! I want to give up or run away." Temporarily feeling overwhelmed is a natural response.

Coping Despite Feeling Overwhelmed

Accept that it is normal to feel this way and that this feeling may come and go. Don't wait to feel better before acting. Take action first. The more active steps you take, the less overwhelmed you will feel. Changing your actions will help change your feelings.

Here are some coping tips:

- If you feel that you face an overwhelming task, break it down into a series of doable steps. Take one small step at a time.

- Talk to other people who are coping well. Join a support group and seek out inspiring examples.

- Read about lymphedema and about managing emotions. Find helpful web sites, like www.LymphNotes.com.

- Periodically take a deliberate break from lymphedema and immerse yourself in pleasurable, distracting activities. Then return to the task of coping with your lymphedema and dealing with your emotional reactions.

Feeling Overwhelmed: Warning Signs

Feeling overwhelmed is not a normal reaction when it stops being temporary or when it leads you to make unhealthy decisions.

Here are some warning signs:

- You are passive. You wait for others to take care of you. You act helpless, useless, or incompetent.

- You don't protect yourself or your body.

- You skip your self-management, miss treatment or medical appointments, or don't take your medication as prescribed.

- You don't ask questions, seek information, or problem-solve.

- You are not physically active.

- You abuse alcohol, drugs, or medications.

These warning signs may also be signs of depression or of other problems discussed above. As always, if you notice these signs, consider consulting a professional.

Summary

In this chapter, I have presented an overview of the common emotional challenges accompanying lymphedema, given you some tips on coping with each normal reaction, and reviewed some of the warning signs that an emotional reaction has become problematic.

I wish you success in coping with the emotional challenges of lymphedema and congratulate you on reading this book. I encourage you to practice emotional coping skills, as well as your lymphedema self-management, and to continue to learn what works for you.

Remember that no matter how difficult the challenges are, the more knowledge and skill you have, the better you can cope. Take care of yourself.

Stories of Lymph Notes Members

- When I was 13, my left foot started to swell. I'm 22 now and having it through all these years when girls are self-conscious was really hard. I wish they would find a cure for this.

- Breast cancer was tough, of course, but there was so much information and understanding. With this "for life" business and the daily maintenance, it is not surprising that I am depressed.

- I am grateful that my family is so supportive and we put our concerns on the important things in life, the babies. There is a lot of healing in holding a new little person and feeding them. When I start to feel sad about myself, I remember all of my children are healthy and working and all of my grandchildren are healthy and studying hard. That helps me so much.

Self-Management of Lymphedema

> ### *Recommended Reading*
>
> Many self-management activities are based on the unique func-
> tioning of the lymphatic system. The reader is urged to review
> **Section IV—Understanding The Lymphatic System** before con-
> tinuing with this section.

Pam's Story, Part II—On Her Own

Pam was back at the *"Here for You"* lymphedema treatment center again. She said, "Hi!" to her new friend Megan (the teen with the iPod). They had gotten acquainted in the exercise class at the center and Pam learned that Megan has primary lymphedema. Although Pam has secondary lymphedema, their treatment was similar and they found that they had fun exercising together, despite Pam's bandages, Megan's compression garment, and their 15 year age difference.

The businessman Pam had seen previously was in the class too. Although Sam didn't say much about the injuries he had suffered, Pam had read the stories of his heroism as a firefighter in the newspaper. Instead of complaining, Sam went about these exercises with a very definite, *"I'm going to win this one too"* attitude. He also had a great sense of humor and had them all laughing a lot.

Pam won't be coming here as often now that she has completed the initial phase of her treatment. She was thrilled to be out of bandages and into a compression garment for day-time wear. She was also a little nervous about being on her own.

Throughout her treatment Pam had been learning the "self-management" skills that would permit her to manage her lymphedema at home and this was it, her last visit for about six months. She needed to pay close attention to her review session today!

Chapter **9**

Skin, Nail, and Foot Care

An essential part of self-management is taking care of the body's outer barriers against infections. This chapter covers care for skin, nails, and feet and includes a lymphedema specific first aid guide.

Skin Care

Lymphedema causes skin problems, as discussed in Chapter 6. In turn, these skin problems make the symptoms of lymphedema worse. This section describes self-management steps to prevent or minimize these problems.

The Functions of Healthy Skin

Healthy skin is free of scrapes, cuts or open sores. It protects the body by:

- Wrapping the body securely in a flexible protective covering.

- Preventing the entry of disease-producing bacteria.

- Protecting the underlying tissues from injury.

- Preventing the excessive loss of body fluids.

- Maintaining normal body temperatures by sweating and shivering.

The Acid Mantle

The *acid mantle* is a thin protective layer that normally covers the surface of skin. This layer is created by the flow of oil from the pores of the sebaceous glands and water from sweat glands.

The purpose of the acid mantle is to slow the growth of harmful bacteria and fungi on the skin. Unfortunately this protective layer can easily be disrupted by:

• Swelling, fragility, and changes in the skin due to lymphedema.

• Washing the skin with harsh soaps.

• Exposure to the sun, wind, cold, and harsh weather.

Daily Skin Care

The goals of skin care are to maintain the acid mantle and the health of the skin. Effective skin care includes the following steps that should be performed daily:

• Wash with a mild soap or an oil-based body wash. Harsh soaps disrupt the acid mantle and dry the skin.

• Wash gently and thoroughly using warm, not hot, water. Heat increases lymphedema-related swelling and can damage the skin.

• Dry the skin by patting gently, taking particular care to dry within the skin folds. A hair dryer on a very low setting can be used to dry awkward areas or between these folds. Because heat damages lymphedema affected tissues, *never use the hair dryer on a high heat*!

• Moisturize the skin with a non-perfumed low pH moisturizing lotion to help maintain the acid mantle and keep the skin flexible to avoid cracking. Many therapists recommend Eucerin Original lotion.

- Examine the affected skin daily, checking for cracks or signs of possible infection (see pages 75 and 77).

- If the skin is flaking due to papillomatosis and your therapist has instructed you to do so, very carefully and gently remove the tiny pieces of loose dead skin. Do this only piece-by-piece, not by rubbing, tugging, or picking at dried pieces! Gentle removal of these flakes helps the underlying tissue become healthier. Removing flakes that are not loose can tear the skin and create an opening for bacteria to enter and cause an infection.

Skin Protection

- Protect against sunburn by wearing a high sun protection factor (SPF) sunscreen when outdoors. Lymphedema-affected skin is very sensitive to the sun and a compression garment does not protect against UV rays.

- Do not permit electrolysis on tissues with, or at risk for, lymphedema because this increases the risk of infection by causing breaks in the skin. *Electrolysis* is the use of electrical current to destroy unwanted hair follicles.

- Do not use a depilatory on tissues with, or at risk for, lymphedema because this can damage the skin. A *depilatory* is a chemical used to remove unwanted hair.

- Do not perform exfoliation on tissues with, or at risk for, lymphedema because this can damage the skin. *Exfoliation* is the use of a coarse soap or cream to remove the outer layer of dead skin cells.

- When gardening or involved in outdoor activities such as walking in the woods wear appropriate protective clothing, such as long sleeves and gloves.

- Pets can be a great joy but any scratch or bite carries the risk of infection. Wear protective clothing or stay away from pets that scratch.

- Pet feces contain bacteria and parasites that can cause infections in humans. Those with lymphedema of the hand or arm should always wear gloves when cleaning the litter box, fish tank or stables; better yet, have someone else take over this responsibility.

- Getting a **tattoo** on lymphedema-affected tissues is not recommended for these reasons: (1) the procedure involves multiple needle sticks with equipment that may not be sterile; (2) 90% of the tattoo dye goes into the nearby lymph nodes and stays there; (3) the tattooed image will be distorted by the lymphedema swelling; and (4) the laser treatments required to remove a tattoo could be harmful to tissues already damaged by lymphedema.

Nail Care

Proper nail care is important because any break in the skin around nails is an invitation to infection. The following guidelines apply to finger or toenails on a limb affected by lymphedema.

- Check daily for any sign of an ingrown nail or an infection around nails. If there are problems in these areas, promptly seek appropriate treatment. Be sure to inform your podiatrist or primary healthcare provider that you have lymphedema.

- Examine between the toes for indications of athlete's foot. The prevention of athlete's foot is discussed in Chapter 6.

- Keep your nails trimmed short and straight across. This helps to reduce the risk of scratching adjacent tissues.

- If you visit a manicurist or pedicurist, be sure that they know that you have lymphedema and are at high risk for infection! Cleanliness is essential and nail care equipment must be sanitized before use. To ensure having clean equipment, you may want to bring your own manicure kit for these visits.

- Do not allow your cuticles to be cut. There is the risk that they may be cut too close, causing a break in the skin that can result in an infection.

- Do not allow the use of chemicals to remove excess cuticle; these destructive chemicals can be absorbed through the skin. One alternative is to soften the cuticle with vegetable oil and to use a clean orange stick to push back the excess tissue. An *orange stick* is a disposable wood implement with tapered ends that is used in manicuring.

- Avoid artificial nails; these nails frequently cause fungal nail infections even in individuals without lymphedema. They also harbor bacteria and this increases the risk of even the smallest scratch becoming infected.

- Dark colored nail polish is best avoided because the area under the polished nails is a warm, dark, and damp environment that increases the risk of a fungal infection.

- Avoid acetone in nail polish removers. This chemical can be irritating when absorbed into the skin.

Foot Care

Proper foot care is extremely important for those with lymphedema of the lower extremities, including children. The primary rules for general foot care are:

- Whenever you are walking or moving around, always have your feet properly supported and protected from injury.

- Do not walk barefoot outdoors or in public places where there is a higher risk of injury or exposure to athlete's foot.

- Always wear properly fitted socks and footwear when walking or hiking in areas where your feet might be cut or scraped. Sandals do not provide adequate protection for "at risk" feet.

Proper Footwear

Properly fitted shoes are a good investment because they help to prevent foot problems (Figure 9-1). They also make you more comfortable, increase your mobility, and help you get the exercise that is so important. When your leg is affected by lymphedema, the following are important factors in selecting shoes:

- Shop for shoes at the time of the day when your foot is most swollen. For most people this is toward the end of the day.

- Wear your compression garment when shopping for shoes. Your shoes must comfortably accommodate this garment.

- Do not compromise on the fit, even if it means that you must buy shoes of two different sizes! You need shoes that are long and wide enough to accommodate your feet without pinching or rubbing. Shoelaces or Velcro® straps will allow you to adjust the fit as your feet change size during the day.

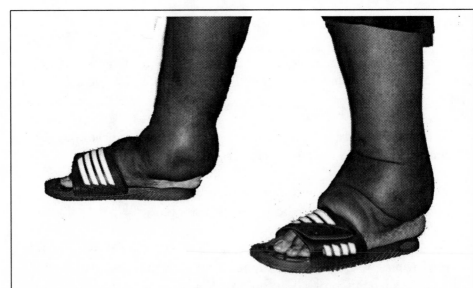

Figure 9-1: The footwear shown here does not fit properly, does not protect the feet, and does not provide adequate support.

- Properly fitting athletic shoes are usually your best choice. They have a wide toe box and are designed to provide good foot support and protection. Shoes with mesh tops allow help keep your feet cool and dry.

- Avoid sandals or open-toed shoes unless they provide proper foot support and protection against injury.

- If you wear orthotics, place them in the shoes you are trying on. *Orthotics* are inserts, such as inner soles or arch supports, that are placed in shoes to improve your ability to walk properly. These can be purchased over-the-counter or custom made based on a prescription from your foot doctor.

- Diabetic shoes may meet your shoe needs because they come in larger and wider sizes, are made of a breathable material, and have a soft lining.

Foot Surgery

Chemical based corn or callus removal pads should never be used on a foot affected by lymphedema due to the risk of burns and infection. Instead, corns or calluses should be treated by a podiatrist, chiropodist, or other healthcare professional. When foot surgery is necessary, follow these precautions:

- Check with your lymphedema therapist in preparation for surgery. Additional MLD sessions may be recommended to maximize the health of these tissues before surgery. Also ask your therapist about wearing your compression garments and aids after surgery.

- Check with your physician, he or she may recommend antibiotics before and after the procedure as a precautionary measure and/or an anti-inflammatory post-operatively to control swelling.

- Check with your lymphedema therapist and your foot specialist to see how soon you can resume MLD treatment to speed healing.

Lymphedema Specific First Aid

Note: this section provides lymphedema specific first aid tips for minor injuries. This guide is not a substitute for professional medical advice or formal first aid training. If you have a medical emergency, or if you are not sure if an injury is serious, call 911 or your local emergency medical assistance number and let them evaluate the injury.

The minor cuts, bumps, and scratches that are part of everyday life are not necessarily a medical crisis for those with, or at risk for, lymphedema. These minor injuries do require prompt treatment with appropriate first aid procedures.

After you have treated the injury, continue to check frequently for indication of infection throughout the healing stage. If any symptoms of infection develop (see pages 75 and 77), seek medical treatment immediately.

When there are no signs of infection, continue with the self-management phase of your lymphedema treatment, including wearing your compression garments and aids. If you have any doubts about this, check with your lymphedema therapist.

First Aid Steps

Despite all precautions, minor accidents involving the affected limb do occur. When managing these events it is important to remember that lymphedema-affected tissues do not recover as quickly as normal tissues do. Therefore, even a minor injury is likely to take longer to heal.

When an accident happens, first carefully follow basic first aid procedures. Then follow these additional guidelines for treating any injury that slightly damages or breaks the skin in the lymphedema-affected area. If your physician has prescribed preventative antibiotics, follow the instructions provided by your doctor.

Minor Cuts or Scratches

- Bleeding helps to clean out wounds, and most small cuts or scrapes will stop bleeding after a short time. If the bleeding does not stop in a timely manner, seek medical care.

- Carefully clean the wound with mild antibacterial soap and water. Hydrogen peroxide is no longer recommended for cleaning wounds.

- Apply an over-the-counter topical antibiotic cream, such as Neosporin.® Note: Some physicians *do not* recommend using antibiotic cream for this purpose, check with your doctor in advance.

- Place a sterile bandage, such as a band-aid, over the wound. For very sensitive skin, use Duoderm® or another brand of skin dressing. If tape cannot be tolerated, place gauze pads and cover them with rolled gauze that is taped to itself.

- Watch for signs of infection! In lymphedema-affected tissues, even a very small wound can lead to a major infection.

Bruises

- If the bruise is on or near a lymphedema-affected limb, examine the injured area carefully to determine that it is only a bruise with no break in the skin. If the skin is broken, treat this injury as a cut or scratch.

- To reduce swelling and minimize discoloration, immediately place a cold pack on the injury. Keep this in place for no longer than 20 minutes at a time.

- The standard recommendation for treating bruises includes alternating ice and heat for the next 48 hours; however, since heat is not recommended on lymphedema-affected tissues, this step should be modified to alternate cold with mild to moderate warmth.

Itchy Rashes

Warning: If you have itching that is not caused by an outside substance, this could be a symptom of erysipelas and require prompt medical treatment (see page 77).

- The first rule of dealing with an itchy rash, such as poison ivy, is *"Don't scratch!!"*

- Treat the rash by cleaning the area and gently applying an antibiotic cream. If blisters are present, do not break them.

- Over-the-counter anti-itch ointments containing hydrocortisone may help relieve the itching.

- If the itching is severe, seek medical help.

- Watch for trouble! The irritants that are producing the rash may cause increased swelling in the affected area and there is always the possibility of an infection.

Insect Bites or Stings

When an insect bites or stings, it injects a toxin into the skin and these toxins cause the resulting itching. A *toxin* is a harmful or poisonous substance. The reaction to insect bites or stings in lymphedema-affected tissues can be severe. There may be a temporary increase in the swelling of the affected limb in response. Also, it may take the body longer than usual to clear the toxins from lymphedema-affected tissues.

- If you have multiple bites on an affected limb, a history of allergic reactions to insects, or you think the insect may be poisonous, seek medical help immediately.

- Don't scratch!! A cool wet cloth will ease the itching and swelling.

- An insect bite is a break in the skin and it should be treated as such. Anti-itch ointments, such as Cortaid®, may help ease the discomfort. If the itching is severe, seek medical help.

- Always pay close attention for signs of trouble or infection!

- As long as no infection is present, it should be safe to perform self-massage to help the body clear toxins from this area.

Burns

Evaluate the extent of damage, and act accordingly:[1]

- **Third degree burns** involve all layers of the skin, fat, muscle, and even bone, the area may be charred black or dry and white. Call 911, make sure the person is breathing (do CPR if necessary), and cover the burn with a cool moist sterile bandage or clean cloth. This type of burn, particularly on lymphedema-affected tissues, requires immediate medical treatment.

- **Second degree burns** damage the first and second layers of skin, blisters develop and the skin takes on a reddened, splotchy, or wet appearance. If the burned area is larger than 2 inches in diameter or includes the hands, feet, face, groin, buttocks, or a major joint, get medical help immediately; minor burns can be treated as described on the next page. Watch closely for any indication of breaking blisters and/or infection because these require prompt medical treatment.

- **First degree burns** redden and damage the outer layer of skin. If the burned area includes the hands, feet, face, groin, buttocks, or a major joint, get medical help immediately. Minor burns can be treated as described on the next page.

Minor burn treatment

Extra caution should be taken when dealing with a burn on lymphedema-affected tissues. Minor burns can be treated by:

- Cooling the burned area with cool running water or a cold, wet cloth. Do not use ice, ice water, butter, or oil.

- Continuing to apply cold water or the wet cloth for 20 minutes and then remove it for 20 minutes, until the area is pain-free.

- Examining the burned area carefully to check for blistering or breaks in the skin. If these are present, seek medical care promptly.

- Applying an antibiotic cream, aloe vera lotion, or a low pH moisturizer over the burn to prevent the burned tissue from drying out.

- Covering the burn loosely with a sterile gauze bandage.

- Taking an anti-inflammatory drug such as aspirin, ibuprofen (Advil, Motrin), naproxen (Aleve), or acetaminophen (Tylenol).

Chapter 10

Self-Massage

The primary purpose of self-massage, also known as *lymphatic massage*, is to improve the flow and drainage of lymph by stimulating the lymphatic vessels. Your lymphedema therapist will instruct you in a program of daily self-massage. This is an important part of managing your lymphedema and should be performed regularly as directed.

However, if you have an infection, or any indication that you are developing an infection, you may need to modify or skip your self-massage until the infection is under control.

Ask First

Check with your physician and lymphedema therapist before beginning a program of self-massage.

Self-massage is not recommended for those with some medical conditions such as certain malignant tumors, leukemia, acute inflammation, tuberculosis, toxoplasmosis, acute allergic reactions, erysipelas, thrombosis, precancerous skin conditions, chronic inflammation, thyroid disorders, bronchial asthma, dysautonomia, granulomas, or occlusive artery disease.

Self-Massage Terminology

Refer to Figure 10-1 and the figures in Section IV for locations:

- The **terminus** is the slight triangular indentation on each side of the base of the neck. It is formed by the clavicle (collarbone) in the front, the neck on the side, and the top of the shoulder muscle at the back.

- The **cervical lymph nodes** are located on the sides of the neck.

- The **axillary lymph nodes** are located under the arms.

- The **inguinal lymph nodes** are located in the groin.

- The **midline** divides the body from top to bottom into equal left and right halves.

- Four **quadrants of the trunk** are created by dividing the trunk into halves with the midline and into fourths with a transverse line through the waist.

- The **affected side** or **affected limb** is the limb or portion of the trunk where the lymphedema swelling occurs.

- The **unaffected side** or **unaffected limb**, also known as the intact side or limb is the area that *is not* affected by lymphedema.

Understanding the Self-Massage Strokes

To understand the self-massage strokes, pay close attention as your therapist performs manual lymph drainage (MLD) during your treatment session. The same sequence and similar strokes are used in self-massage. Self-massage is an important part of self-management; however, it does not replace MLD treatments provided by a trained lymphedema therapist.

Figure 10-1: Important terms related to self-massage.

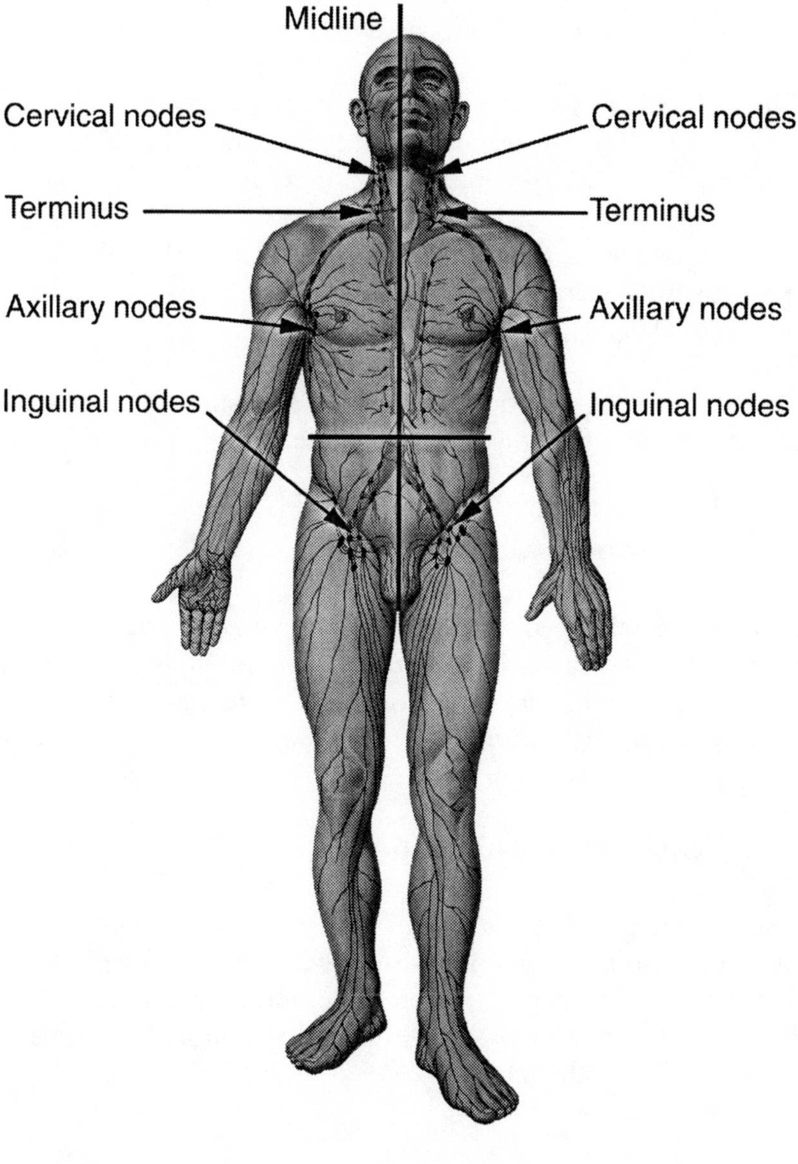

Midline

Cervical nodes   Cervical nodes

Terminus   Terminus

Axillary nodes   Axillary nodes

Inguinal nodes   Inguinal nodes

- Self-massage is a gentle technique that should never hurt or make the skin red.[1]

- Self-massage to encourage lymph drainage *is not* the same as conventional muscle massage. It is important not to allow anyone, other than a trained lymphedema therapist, to massage you using deep strokes.

- Most self-massage strokes use very little pressure and the hands do not slide over the skin. Instead they move and stretch the skin to stimulate the lymphatic capillaries located just under the skin.

- Oils and lotions that make the skin slippery *are not used* during self massage. If the skin is very dry, lotion may be applied and allowed to be absorbed before beginning the massage.

- When massaging fibrotic tissues, use the pressure and strokes recommended by your therapist to soften these hardened tissues.

Rhythmic Pumping Motion

A rhythmic pumping self-massage motion is used to stimulate areas such as the terminus and major lymph nodes. This motion is performed by very gently pressing with the fingers, moving the skin in a circle the size of a coin, and then releasing the pressure.

Stretch-Twist-Release Motion

The stretch-twist-release motion is used to stimulate the flow of lymph through the skin. This motion is performed by gently placing three fingers on the skin. The fingers gently stretch the skin for about an inch (2.5 cm) without sliding and then twist slightly to the right and left. This stroke is completed by lifting the fingers.

Sweeping Motion

A sweeping motion, known as *effleurage*, is used at the conclusion of a massage as a final stimulation of the lymph flow through the skin. This motion is performed as a gentle sweep of the fingers across the skin, as if brushing bread crumbs from a table.

Overview of Self-Massage

The information provided here will help you remember the sequence and strokes your therapist has instructed you to use. It is also a helpful guide for a caregiver or helper who is assisting you with self-massage. You will find it beneficial to review the description of the lymphatic system in Section IV while learning self-massage.

The Rhythm of Flowing Lymph

The subtle pumping motion of the lymphatic vessels moves the lymph upward toward the terminus in a rhythm of five-to-seven pulsations per minute.[2] To match these pulsations, each self-massage movement should be repeated from five-to-seven times in the same position. By following this pattern, you enhance the effectiveness of your self-massage as you work with the natural pattern of the flow of lymph.

Preparing for the Flow of Lymph

As explained in Section IV, lymph flows from the tips of the extremities toward the trunk. Within the trunk, lymph flows upward to the terminus where it returns to the venous blood circulation via the subclavian veins.

In contrast to this pattern of flow, self-massage begins with the terminus and moves down to clear the major groups of lymph nodes and the trunk. The final area to be massaged is the affected limb. This massage sequence clears space within the lymphatic ducts to receive the lymph as it flows out of the affected limb or area.

The axillary and inguinal lymph nodes give the greatest resistance to the flow of lymph and these nodes must be cleared before, during, and after massaging the limbs. If these nodes overfill after they have been cleared, they can feel hard and sore. If this happens, clear the terminus and then clear these lymph node groups again, to make room for lymph as it drains from the impaired area.

Which Areas Should You Massage?

Your therapist will design a self-massage program for you that takes into account the parts of your body that are affected by lymphedema, plus the condition of the skin in each of these areas and any other medical conditions or special needs that you may have.

Self-Massage Guidelines, shown on the next page, will help you determine which areas to massage and the massage sequence, based on the parts of your body that are affected. To use this table:

- Highlight the column corresponding to your affected areas.

- Follow the instructions and notes to find the areas you should self-massage. Perform your self-massage in the sequence shown in the table.

Preparing for Self-Massage

Select a room for your self-massage that is quiet and at a comfortable temperature. Perform your massage in the positions that work best for you. Most commonly this is lying on your back in a comfortable and relaxed position. You may want to remove your glasses, jewelry, and any restrictive clothing.

Each self-massage begins with a few quiet moments of deep breathing to help you relax and focus on the task at hand. This breathing pattern, which is discussed in Chapter 12, should be maintained throughout the massage session.

Self-Massage Guidelines

Areas to Massage	Affected Area(s):					
	Head	Arm	Chest	Abdomen	Genital	Leg
Terminus	Yes	Yes	Yes	Yes	Yes	Yes
Head & Neck	Yes	Yes	Yes	Yes	Yes	Yes
Axillary Nodes	Yes	Yes	**	Yes	Yes	Yes
Inguinal Nodes	Yes	Yes	Yes	Yes	Yes	Yes
Midline		Yes	Yes	***		***
Lower Chest			***	***	***	***
Abdomen		Yes	Yes	Yes	Yes	Yes
Affected Arm		Yes	Yes			
Affected Leg			Yes	Yes	***	Yes
Upper Back		Yes	Yes	Yes	Yes	Yes
Lower Back				Yes	***	Yes

** If both sides of the chest are affected, do not massage the axillary area.

*** Optional: Check with your therapist.

Self-massage is best performed first thing in the morning, before bandaging or exercising, and at other times as specified by your therapist.

The length of time devoted to self-massage depends on your condition and the instructions provided by your therapist. Most people find that self-massage only takes a few minutes.

> *If your therapist provides a different self-massage routine, follow the directions given by your therapist*

The Terminus is the Starting Point

Some people can massage the terminus on both sides at once by crossing their arms as shown in Figure 10-2; others find it more comfortable to do one side at a time.

1. Stimulate the terminus by placing your fingers within the indentation at the base of the neck. Use a rhythmic pumping motion as your fingers make a coin-size circle moving toward the back and coming forward toward the midline. Release the pressure as you move your fingers beyond the midline.

2. Repeat this pattern five to seven times.

The Head and Neck

1. Stimulate the cervical lymph nodes by placing your fingers flat along the side of the neck. Move your fingers in a gentle stretch-twist-release motion. Stretch the skin upward, twist toward the back, and release in a downward motion. Repeat these motions moving progressively down the neck. You may be able to

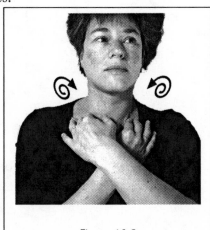

Figure 10-2

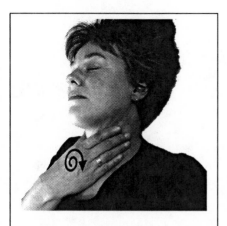

Figure 10-3

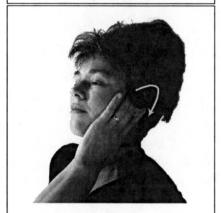

Figure 10-4

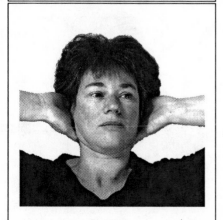

Figure 10-5

do both sides at once or one side at a time as shown in Figure 10-3.

2. Stimulate the lymph nodes near the ears and jaw by massaging the region in front of and behind each ear (see Figure IV-3). On each side of the head, place the thumb and index finger behind the ear with the remaining fingers in front of the ear and the palm of the hand on the cheek. Slowly and gently make a stretch-twist-release motion. Move the skin upward, twisting toward the back, and release in a downward motion (Figure 10-4).

3. Stimulate the lymph nodes at the base of the skull by placing your fingers behind the ears with the base of the hands resting on the back of the lower jaw. With the finger tips, slowly and gently make a stretch-twist-release motion. Move the skin upward, twist toward the back, and release in a downward motion toward the ears (Figure 10-5).

Clearing the Axillary Nodes

There are two clusters of axillary nodes: one at the front of the armpit under the pectoral muscle of the chest, and another at the rear of the armpit under the latissimus dorsi muscle of the back.

If the chest area is involved, as after breast cancer, clear only on the unaffected side. If both sides of the chest are affected, do not massage the axillary area. Instead clear only on the neck and lower quadrants, or proceed as instructed by your therapist.

Clearing the Front Axillary Nodes

1. To clear the front axillary nodes use light pressure with a gentle rhythmic pumping motion.

2. Place your fingers gently on the skin in the armpit behind the pectoral muscle.

3. Make slow circular pumping motions with the finger tips. Move the fingers into the armpit and then upward toward the trunk (Figure 10-6).

4. Maintain skin contact as you release the pressure and then move the fingers away.

Clearing the Back Axillary

Nodes

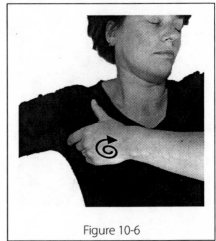

Figure 10-6

1. To clear the back axillary nodes use light pressure with a gentle rhythmic pumping motion.

2. Place your fingers gently on the skin in the armpit in front of the latissimus dorsi muscle of the back.

3. Make slow circular pumping motions with the fingertips. Move the fingers into the armpit and then upward toward the trunk.

4. Maintain skin contact as you release the pressure and then move the fingers away.

Clearing the Inguinal Nodes

The inguinal lymph nodes are located in the lower groin where the legs meet the trunk (see Figure IV-10). These nodes are massaged from the leg toward the trunk using slightly more pressure than on the axillary nodes.

1. Place your hands gently on the skin of the upper thigh, just below the crease of the groin.

2. Use your whole hand to make a rhythmic circular pumping action slowly and gently with the pressure directed upward toward the trunk (Figure 10-7).

3. Maintain skin contact as you release the pressure and then move your hand away.

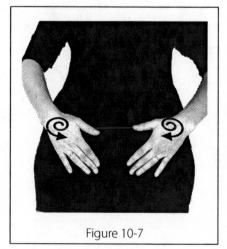

Figure 10-7

Clearing Across the Midline

Clearing across the midline encourages the flow of lymph from the affected (damaged) side into the unaffected (intact) side where the lymph can be collected and transported to the terminus.

If both sides are affected do not clear across the midline.

If the axillary nodes on both sides are intact, clear across the midline on each side.

If the axillary nodes on one side are affected, clear only from the affected side onto the unaffected side.

Do not clear from the unaffected side onto the affected side. Doing this increases the amount of lymph to be handled by the already damaged lymphatics of the affected side.

Clearing Across the Midline from the Affected Side

Note: Instructions and illustrations in this section are based on an affected **right** side.

1. Place the right hand flat on the affected side with the fingers slightly spread just below the throat. Slide the hand gently to the left across the midline with an upward swing toward the terminus on the left side of the neck (Figure 10-8).

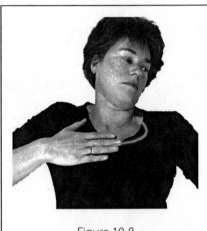

Figure 10-8

2. Move the starting position of the hand downward toward the waist and repeat these sliding motions across the midline to the axillary nodes in the left armpit (Figure 10-9).

Self-Massage Between the Ribs

There are many small lymph nodes located in the space between the ribs. This self-massage step moves the lymph gently downward into these nodes.

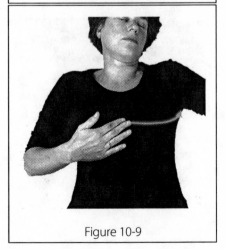

Figure 10-9

1. Place the fingers of the right hand flat against the ribs on the affected side.

2. Make a gentle pumping and release motion in the space between the ribs.

Self-Massage of the Lower Chest

Self-massage of the lower chest is used to ease swelling or tenderness in the chest region or if there is swelling, tenderness, and a feeling of fullness in the upper abdomen. If your therapist wants you to include the lower chest in your self-massage, he or she will tell you at what stage in your self-massage these steps should be included.

Continue your relaxed deep breathing throughout this massage.

1. Place the palm of one hand on top of the other over your stomach in the area where the ribs join the breastbone.

2. As you breathe in, let your hands follow the breathing. Then gently push down as you breathe out. *Caution:* To avoid damaging the lower tip of the breastbone, do not use much pressure here.

3. Place your hands just above the navel and make a gentle upward sweeping movement toward the unaffected side.

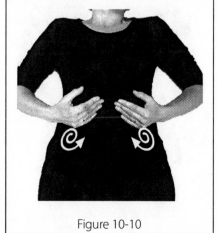

Figure 10-10

4. Place the hands just below the edge of the rib cage on each side of the chest. Make a deep, but gentle, circular pumping action upward into these tissues (Figure 10-10).

5. Repeat clearing the axillary lymph nodes on the unaffected side and then repeat clearing the terminus.

Self-Massage of the Abdomen

Self-massage of the abdomen clears and stimulates the larger lymphatic structures located in this area. It also stimulates the flow of lymph through the many nodes located near the intestines (see Figure IV- 9).

In preparation for clearing the abdomen, empty the bladder to prevent accidental leakage during the deep massage. This also prepares the bladder to receive the additional fluid excreted by the kidneys.

Abdominal Self-Massage

Perform abdominal self-massage while lying in a relaxed position.

1. Place the palm of one hand on top of the other over your navel. Breathe deeply so that your stomach raises—not your chest. As you breathe out, your stomach will flatten (Figure 10-11). As you breathe in, gently scoop upwards with your hands to create a mild pressure in the pelvic region. Release the pressure as you breathe out.

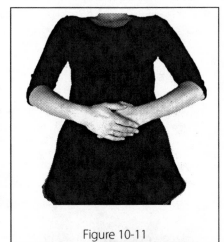

Figure 10-11

2. With each new breath, gradually move your hands down toward the pubic bone. Repeat this pressure/release hand movement pattern until you reach the top of the pubic bone.

3. Place the palm of one hand on top of the other in the lower right corner of your abdomen (Figure 10-12). As you breathe in, make a slow,

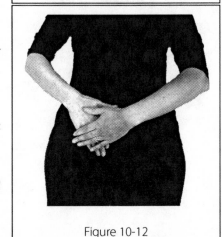

Figure 10-12

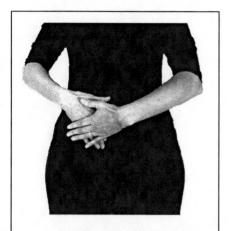

Figure 10-13

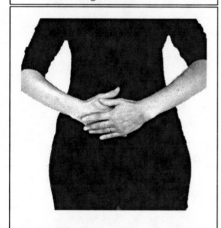

Figure 10-14

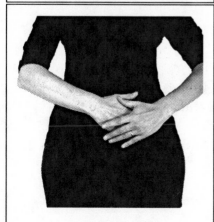

Figure 10-15

gentle, rhythmic pumping motion downward toward the pubic bone. Release with an upward motion toward the navel and then breathe out. This is the beginning of a clockwise series of motions that follows the right-to-left flow of the bowel.

4. Move your hands up toward the waist about two inches (5 cm), and repeat these motions as you slowly breathe in (Figure 10-13). Release with an upward motion toward the navel and then breathe out.

5. Move your hands up and left, about two inches (5 cm) toward the midline, and repeat these motions as you slowly breathe in (Figure 10-14). Release toward the navel and then breathe out.

6. Move your hands to the left, across the midline, and repeat these motions as you slowly breathe in (Figure 10-15). Release toward the groin, then breathe out.

7. Move your hands progressively down the left side of the abdomen. Repeat these motions as you slowly breathe in (see Figure 10-16). Release toward the groin, then breathe out.

8. Finish these motions in the left corner of the abdomen, across from the starting point.

9. Complete this portion of the self-massage by clearing the inguinal lymph nodes again.

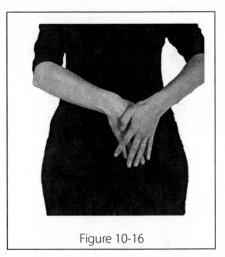

Figure 10-16

Arm Self-Massage

The self-massage of the arm always begins near the body, moves downward to the fingers, and then moves upward again toward the trunk. If both arms are affected, ask your therapist which arm should be treated first.

Arm Self-Massage Summary

☐ Clear the terminus.

☐ Massage the head and neck.

☐ Clear the axillary lymph nodes on the unaffected side.

☐ Clear the inguinal lymph nodes.

☐ Clear across the midline from the affected side to the unaffected side.

☐ Massage the abdomen.

☐ Massage the affected arm starting from the shoulder: upper arm, elbow, lower arm, wrist, hand and fingers.

☐ Massage the affected arm starting from the fingertips: hand and fingers, wrist, lower arm, elbow, and upper arm.

☐ Repeat massage of the abdomen, inguinal, unaffected axillary lymph nodes, and the terminus.

Unaffected Arm Self-Massage

Your therapist may recommend self-massage of the unaffected arm to clear the lymphatics in that area. If so, this arm is always massaged before proceeding to the affected arm. Self-massage of the unaffected arm uses the same techniques and sequence as those used when massaging the affected arm.

Affected Arm Self-Massage

The illustrations shown in this section are for the self-massage of an affected **left** arm.

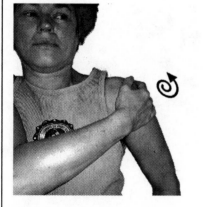

Figure 10-17

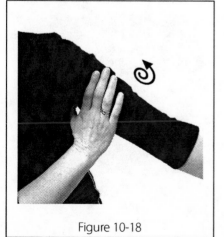

Figure 10-18

1. Continue deep breathing during the massage of the affected arm.

2. On the outer surface of the upper arm, use the stretch-twist-release motion to stretch upward and twist toward the back of the shoulder. Repeat this pattern in three locations, moving progressively down the upper arm toward the elbow (Figure 10-17).

3. On the inner surface of the upper arm, use the stretch-twist-release motion to stretch toward the outside and twist toward the back of the shoulder. Repeat this pattern in three locations, moving progressively down the upper arm toward the elbow (Figure 10-18).

4. In the bend of the elbow, make a gentle rhythmic pump-and-release motion (Figure 10-19).

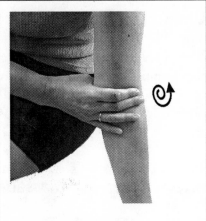

Figure 10-19

5. On the inner surface of the forearm, use the stretch-twist-release motion to stretch upward and twist toward the back of the arm. Repeat this pattern in three locations moving progressively down the forearm toward the wrist (Figure 10-20).

6. On the outer surface of the forearm, gently use the stretch-twist-release motion to stretch upward and twist toward the elbow. Repeat this pattern in three locations, moving progressively down toward the wrist.

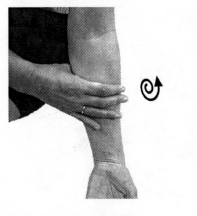

Figure 10-20

7. At the wrist, make stationary circles using a pump-and-release motion (Figure 10-21).

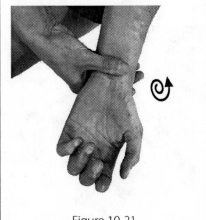

Figure 10-21

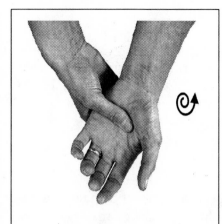

Figure 10-22

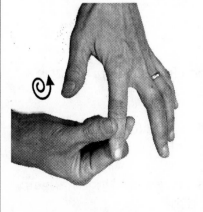

Figure 10-23

8. On the palm and back of the hand, make stationary circles using a pump and release motion (Figures 10-22 and 10-23).

9. On each finger and thumb, starting at the base and working towards the tip, make circular motions toward the base (Figure 10-24). If you notice that the increased drainage has filled the axillary nodes, repeat clearing the terminus and the axillary nodes.

10. Finish with a light sweeping stroke from your fingertips up your arm to the back of the shoulder (Figure 10-25). As shown in this figure, the arm is being supported against the leg.

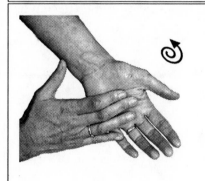

Figure 10-24

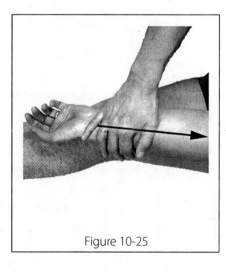

Figure 10-25

Leg Self-Massage

The self-massage of the leg always begins near the body, moves downward to the toes, and then moves upward again toward the trunk. If both legs are affected, ask your therapist which should be treated first.

Unaffected Leg Self-Massage

Your therapist may recommend including self-massage of the unaffected leg to clear the lymphatics in that area. If so, this leg is always massaged before proceeding to the affected leg. Self-massage of the unaffected leg uses the same techniques and sequence as those used when treating the affected leg.

Leg Self-Massage Summary

- ☐ Clear the terminus.

- ☐ Self-massage the head and neck.

- ☐ Clear the axillary lymph nodes.

- ☐ Clear the inguinal lymph nodes.

- ☐ Self-massage the abdomen.

- ☐ Self-massage the affected leg starting from the hip: upper leg, knee, lower leg, ankle, foot and toes.

- ☐ Self-massage the affected leg starting from the toes: foot and toes, ankle, lower leg, knee, and upper leg.

- ☐ Self-massage the abdomen, clear the unaffected inguinal lymph nodes, the axillary lymph nodes, and the terminus.

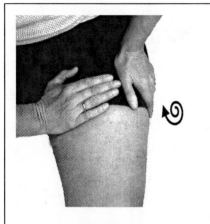

Figure 10-26

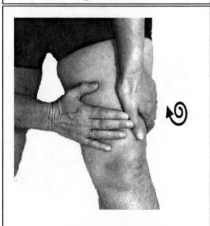

Figure 10-27

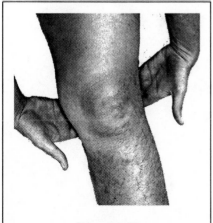

Figure 10-28

Affected Leg Self-Massage

The illustrations in this section show the massage of an affected **left** leg.

1. Starting on the outer surface at the top of the thigh, use the stretch-twist-release motion to stretch upward and twist toward the back of the hip (Figure 10-26). Release the pressure of your fingers upward toward the hip. Repeat this motion in progressively lower positions until you reach the knee.

2. On the inner surface of the thigh, starting near the hip, use the stretch-twist-release motion to stretch upward and twist toward the outer surface of the leg with an upward pressure toward the hip (Figure 10-27). Release the pressure of your fingers upward toward the hip. Repeat this motion in progressively lower positions until you reach the knee.

3. In the back of the bend of the knee, make a gentle rhythmic pumping action with a release towards the front of the knee (Figure 10-28).

4. On the front of the knee, make a circular pump-and-release motion moving in and up towards the trunk (Figure 10-29).

5. On the outer surface of the lower leg, use the stretch-twist-release motion to stretch upward, twist toward the outer surface of the leg and release the pressure of your fingers toward the knee.

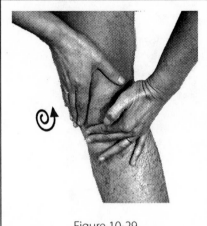

Figure 10-29

6. On the inner surface of the lower leg below the knee, use the stretch-twist-release motion to stretch upward, twist toward the outer surface of the leg with an upward pressure toward the knee and release the pressure of your fingers. Repeat this motion in progressively lower positions until you reach the ankle (Figure 10-30).

7. On the ankle, perform stationary circles with your thumbs (Figure 10-31).

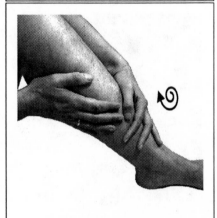

Figure 10-30

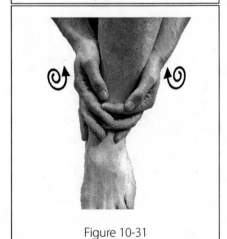

Figure 10-31

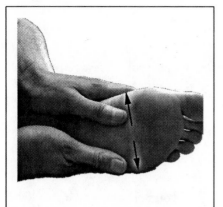

Figure 10-32

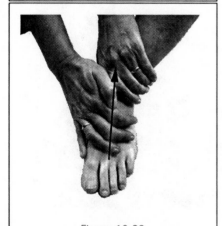

Figure 10-33

8. On the sole of the foot, starting at the heel, use your thumbs to stretch the skin gently from the midline of the sole toward the edges of the foot. Repeat moving up the foot to the toes (Figure 10-32).

9. On the top of the foot, stroke gently upward toward the ankle (Figure 10-33).

10. On your toes, make circular motions from the tip of the toes toward the base (Figure 10-34).

11. Finish with a light sweeping stroke from the foot up the leg to the groin area (Figure 10-35).

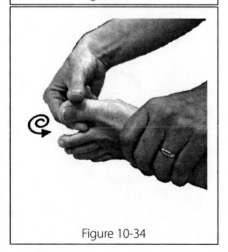

Figure 10-34

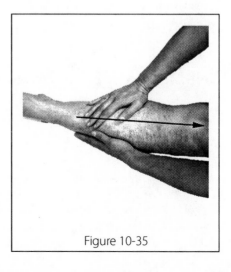

Figure 10-35

Massage of the Back

Massaging your own back is difficult but can be helpful. Massage by a caregiver is more effective, especially in relieving accumulated lymph around the waist.

Self-Massage of the Upper Back

Parts of your back can be reached by hugging yourself or by working with one arm at a time. Massage the parts of your back that you can reach, starting from your waist and working up to the axillary area using a gentle rhythmic pump and release motion (Figure 10-36).

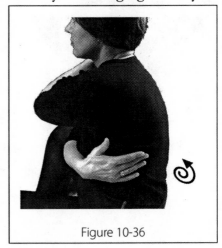

Another way in which to self-massage the back is through the use of a bath towel. Drape the towel across the back. On the affected side, hold one end of the towel up over the shoulder. On the unaffected side, use the other hand to hold the towel near the waist. Gentle downward movement of the towel causes the skin to move and this stimulates the flow of lymph toward the unaffected side.

Figure 10-36

Self-Massage of the Lower Back

This self-massage is done while lying on your stomach or standing.

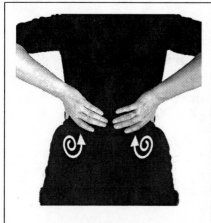

Figure 10-37

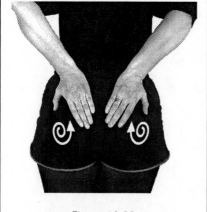

Figure 10-38

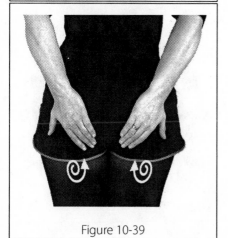

Figure 10-39

1. Place your hands on your waist at the back with the fingers pointing towards the tailbone. Make a gentle circular pump and release motion up towards the head (Figure 10-37).

2. Place the hands flat on your upper buttocks. Make a gentle pump and release motion up towards the head (Figure 10-38).

3. Place the hands flat on the cheeks of the buttocks. Make a gentle pump and release motion up towards the head (Figure 10-39).

Massage of the Upper Back by a Helper

These instructions are guidelines for the helper who is performing manual lymph drainage on your upper back. There are many possible variations of these techniques and it is important that your lymphedema therapist teach your helper the strokes that are appropriate for your treatment.

Two versions are given below. Use the first version when both sets of axillary nodes are intact. Use the second version when the axillary nodes on one side are affected. If the axillary nodes on both sides are affected, ask your therapist for specific guidance.

- The person being massaged should lie on his or her stomach with the forehead resting on a pillow or towel and the arms at the sides.

- Massage using light strokes with warm hands and a consistent rhythm.

- The skin may be moisturized before the massage begins; however, oils and lotions that make the skin slippery *are not used during self massage*.

- Try to maintain hand contact at all times by alternating hands and touching lightly while moving hands between locations.

When the Axillary Nodes are Unaffected

1. Starting at the top of the right shoulder blade, place the hand flat on the back and sweep across the midline upward toward the terminus. This motion is similar to the one shown in Figure 10-40.

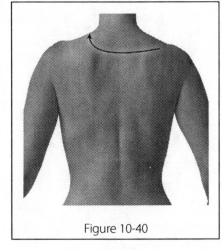

Figure 10-40

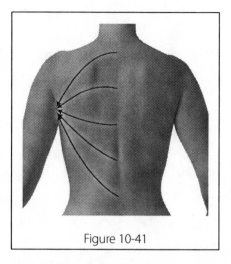

Figure 10-41

2. Starting at the base of the neck, sweep the skin from the spine toward the left axillary node five to seven times (Figure 10-41). Repeat at five different starting points, moving down from the neck toward the waist.

3. Repeat steps one and two on the other side, ending at the right terminus and the right axillary nodes.

When the Axillary Nodes Are Affected

Always go from the affected side to the unaffected side!

When the axillary nodes on only one side are affected, use this technique to clear across the midline of the back from the affected side to the unaffected side. Instructions and illustrations in this section are based on an affected **right** side.

1. Gently massage the axillary nodes at the rear of the unaffected (left) armpit five-to-seven times.

2. Place the whole hand, with the fingers slightly spread, flat on the upper part of the right side of the back with the fingertips near the top of the shoulder blade. Keep the hand flat and slide it gently across the midline, ending with an upward swing toward the terminus on the unaffected side (see Figure 10-40). Gently repeat this motion five-to-seven times.

3. On the right side, sweep the skin
   across the spine toward the left axillary nodes five to seven times. Progressively move the starting point of
   the hand down toward the waist but
   always end at the left axillary nodes
   (Figure 10-42). Perform these
   sweeping strokes from five different
   starting points.

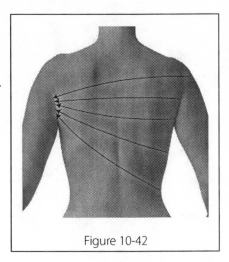

Figure 10-42

Genital Self-Massage

The key to draining the genital area is to clear the axillary and inguinal
lymph nodes to open up space for the lymph from the genital area. Self-
massage of the abdomen is also a very important preparation for moving
lymph through the genital area.

For men it is helpful to elevate the penis and scrotum by placing a folded
towel under the penis and on top of the legs. This takes advantage of the action of gravity during the massage.

Helpful Devices

An easy way to reach more of your back
and body is by using a device that extends your reach. For example, a soft
bath brush with a long handle can be
used to stimulate the skin in hard to
reach areas (Figure 10-43). These gentle brush strokes should not exceed the
pressure you would use when patting a
cat on the back.

Other massage devices such as rods,
bars, or any cylindrical object that rolls
smoothly over the skin can be utilized

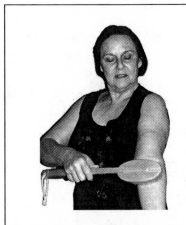

Figure 10-43: A soft bath brush with
a long handle makes it possible to
self-massage places that are not easy
to reach.

to help drain impaired areas. While using such a device, be aware that pressure should be very gentle.[3] Always follow the same patterns and principles of self-massage using your hands.

Scar Massage

Scar tissue can block the flow of lymph. Self-massage to help normalize scar tissue is another important part of managing your lymphedema. Scars from surgery or an injury are treated differently than scars from radiation.

Surgical Scars

Always check with your therapist before beginning scar massage treatment. Scar tissue usually heals within six weeks after surgery but instead of feeling soft and stretchy, a scar may still be red and so tight that it pulls and limits motions.

There are two different approaches to ease scar tissue. The first technique is a gentle circular draining motion on the scar itself. The second is a firmer stretching of the skin above and below the scar, first in a straight line and then in a circular motion.

Gently perform scar massage for five minutes daily.[4] Include all scars that are limiting lymph movement. Stretches use a firm motion but should not cause an uncomfortable pulling or burning sensation. It is important to spend more time on any areas that feel "stuck."

Do not use lotion during scar massage as it causes the fingers to slide. After draining or stretching a scar, apply lotion or vitamin E cream to the scar.

Draining the Scar

Place your fingers on top of the scar and make very gentle circular pumping motions on the scar. Gently work your way down the scar and feel the tissue soften. Repeat this sequence once or twice at each session. This draining of the scar should not hurt nor should it make the scar turn red.

Stretching the Scar Area

To stretch the skin next to the scar, place two or three fingers at the beginning of the scar and stretch the skin above the scar in a parallel direction. Then move the fingers a quarter of an inch (60 mm) further along the scar and repeat the stretch of the adjacent tissue. Work your way along the scar. Repeat this pattern stretching the adjacent skin below the scar.

An alternative method is to follow the same pattern of finger movements using a circular motion instead of straight stretches. Work your way along the scar in a clockwise and counter clockwise fashion.

Radiation Scarring

The scarring processes can continue for as long as six months after the last radiation treatment. Massage of the affected area should not begin until at least six weeks after the last radiation treatment and when no scabs are noticeable. Ask your therapist when you can safely begin self-massage of the radiation scarred areas.

Radiated tissues are delicate and the skin can break easily. Take extreme care when massaging this area. Never massage these tissues if this causes pain or increased redness of the tissues. Perform only brief massage sessions at first. As the tissues continue to heal, gradually increase the length of the massage.

- Move your fingers in a circular motion to gently stretch the skin.

- If there is a pocket of hardened tissue, very gently stretch the skin until the skin feels softer, more flexible, and is less restricting of movements.

- After the massage, apply lotion or vitamin E cream to the scar.

Chapter 11

Self-Bandaging

Self-bandaging is described here to reinforce what your therapist has taught you (or will teach you) and to help you better understand the process.

Self-bandaging is used during the beginning phase of lymphedema treatment. At this time your therapist bandaged the affected limb and taught you, or your caregiver, how to perform self-bandaging. The methods of bandaging vary greatly depending upon the needs of the patient and the techniques in which the therapist has been trained. However, the final goal is the same: to achieve the greatest possible benefit for the patient.

As treatment progresses, some patients are able to replace bandages with a compression garment and/or a compression aid (see Chapter 3). Other patients continue to bandage as part of their self-management program because bandaging is the most effective way for them to reduce swelling, prevent additional swelling, and soften hardened (fibrotic) tissues.

If it is necessary for you to continue self-bandaging, your therapist will instruct you or your caregiver in the techniques to be used. Pay close attention to these instructions and ask questions if a point is not clear because you must be able to follow these instructions exactly each time you bandage at home.

You may want to make a video tape of your therapist demonstrating how to apply your bandages.

Exceptions to Self-Bandaging

☐ Infected areas are not bandaged until after the infection has been treated and brought under control. See signs of infection on pages 75 and 77.

☐ If an open wound is present, check with your therapist for special bandaging precautions.

☐ Certain medical conditions, such as congestive heart failure, do not allow bandaging or require special bandaging. Keep your therapist informed of any changes in your medical condition.

Advance Preparations

1. Gather all necessary materials before you start. Use the supply checklist on the next page or create your own list.

2. Wash and dry your hands.

3. Gently wash and dry the affected limb and inspect it for sores, breaks in the skin, or signs of infection. If you find any of these, they must be treated as instructed by your therapist.

4. Apply a pH-neutral lotion.

Bandaging Basics

• **Bandages should never cause pain, numbness, or discoloration of the fingers or toes.** If these symptoms occur, remove the bandages immediately.

• **Bandaging always begins at the fingers or toes and continues upward toward the body.**[1] This pattern enhances the effectiveness of the bandages because they are following the normal flow of lymph.

Self-Bandaging Supply Checklist

☐ Soap, water, and towels

☐ Low pH moisturizing skin lotion

☐ Scissors

☐ Tubular bandage of the appropriate size

☐ Gauze bandages of the appropriate size

☐ Padding of the appropriate size

☐ Short-stretch bandages for the hand or foot

☐ Short-stretch bandages for the arm or leg

☐ Tape to secure the short-stretch bandages

• **Bandaging usually covers the entire limb all the way to the shoulder or hip.** In some special situations leg bandaging stops just below the knee.

• **Bandages are applied so they are smooth and wrinkle free.** Wrinkled bandages can damage the tissues.

• **Bandages must also be capable of staying in place during exercise and normal activities.** Bandages that slide out of place are annoying, have not been placed properly, and are not working effectively.

• **When bandaging is complete, the pressure is greatest in the finger or toes and the pressure is least nearest the body.** These pressure differences discourage lymph from pooling at the lower end of the extremity.

• **Bandages are never taped to the skin or attached with metal clips.** Metal clips or taping to the skin could cause breaks in the skin that can lead to infections. The end of the last bandage is held in place by a piece of tape that is placed on the top layer of the bandage.

Multilayer Bandaging

Bandages are created from several layers of materials. Each layer has a specific purpose and the layers must be applied in the appropriate sequence.

First Layer: Stockinette

The first layer is a tubular gauze bandage, known as *stockinette*, which is shown in Figure 11-1. This material absorbs excess perspiration and protects the skin from being rubbed by other layers that are placed on top of it.

- For the leg, the stockinette extends from the base of the toes upward as high as you need to bandage.

- For the arm, the stockinette extends from the base of the fingers upward as high on the arm as you need to bandage. Prepare the arm stockinette by making a small cut about an inch from the base of the stockinette. The thumb is placed through this opening to allow for a free range of motion.

- Gently slide the stockinette on the affected limb and smooth it in place.

- A special adhesive solution recommended by your lymphedema therapist may be used to keep the top of the stockinette in place.

- The stockinette is in direct contact with the skin and a fresh piece should be used each time you bandage.

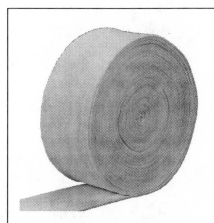

Figure 11-1: Stockinette is the first layer in bandaging.

Second Layer: Gauze

The second layer consists of specialized gauze, which is shown in Figure 11-2. Gauze bandages do not launder well and fresh gauze must be used each time you bandage.

Gauze is wrapped around the individual fingers or toes to reduce and control swelling in these areas. If there is no significant swelling in the fingers or toes, your therapist may instruct you to omit this layer.

- For fingers, one inch gauze is commonly used.

- For toes, one-half inch gauze is commonly used.

As an alternative to gauze, your therapist may suggest specialized short-stretch finger or toe bandages, which can be laundered, or a compression glove.

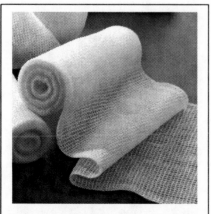

Figure 11-2: Gauze in different widths may be used to wrap fingers or toes.

Third Layer: Protective Padding

The third layer is a felt or foam-type bandage, as shown in Figure 11-3, which is applied to evenly distribute pressure, to soften fibrotic tissues, and to help shape the limb.[2]

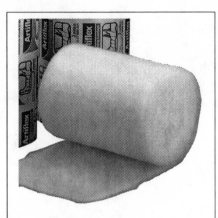

Figure 11-3: Padding is used to help shape the limb and soften fibrotic tissues.

- The protective padding layer is wrapped around the limb as instructed by your therapist (Figure 11-4).

- This layer may be used to hold small, shaped foam pieces in place. These foam pieces protect the indentations (inside of the elbow, front of the ankle, and back of the knee) and prominences (outside of the elbow, front of the knee or back of the ankle) of the limb.

- This layer may be used to hold "chip bags" in place. Chip bags, which contain small irregularly shaped pieces of foam, are placed where needed to soften hardened (fibrotic) tissue.

- Protective padding must be kept clean. 100 percent natural materials such as cotton, flannel, or wool can be laundered easily. For other materials, such as foam, follow the manufacturer's care instructions.

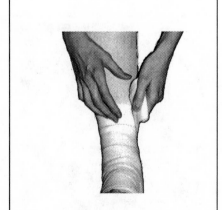

Figure 11-4 Padding is placed over the stockinette. .

Fourth Layer: Short-Stretch Bandages

The fourth layer consists of short-stretch bandages that allow for high working pressure and low resting pressure (Figure 11-5):

- **Working pressure** is caused by the motion of muscles in the bandaged limb while walking or exercising.

- **Resting pressure** is the pressure of the bandage that acts as a counterforce to improve lymphatic function during rest or sleep.

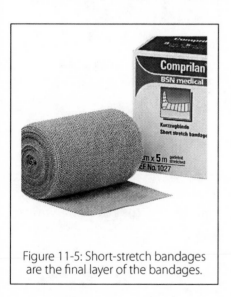

Figure 11-5: Short-stretch bandages are the final layer of the bandages.

Foam Protection

Specially fitted pieces of foam can provide extra protection and comfort. This material is available in sheets that can be cut to the proper size and shape. For example, it can be cut to fit around the lower leg. This foam also creates a shape that is easier to wrap with the short stretch bandages.

An Overview of Short-Stretch Bandage Placement

- Bandaging begins with the fingers or toes. Your therapist may recommend gauze or specialized short-stretch bandages for the fingers or toes.

- Short-stretch bandages are placed to provide greatest compression at the far end of the limb and the least compression near the body (Figure 11-6).

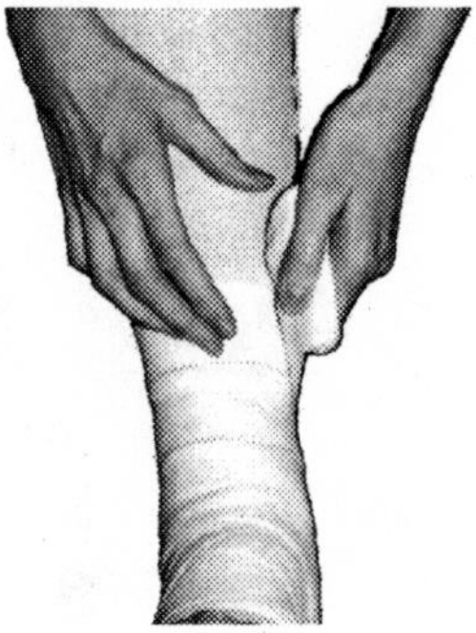

- Usually a smaller width bandage is used for the hand or foot. The higher up the limb, the wider the bandages need to be in order to accommodate the size of the limb.

Figure 11-6: The short-stretch bandages are wrapped smoothly around the limb.

- When all of one roll of bandage has been placed, the end is left flat. This end is secured in place by putting the first turn of the next roll of bandage over the flat last half turn of the previous roll.

- The final roll of bandages is secured to itself by means of tape placed on the bandage.

The Care of Short-Stretch Bandages

Good personal hygiene and clean bandaging materials are essential in maintaining skin health and preventing infections. It is useful to have two sets of short-stretch bandaging materials so that one set can be worn while the other set is being laundered.

- Short-stretch bandages are washed at least once a week to restore their elasticity and cleanliness. If soiled, these bandages should be washed more often.

- These bandages can be washed by hand in lukewarm water using a mild detergent or in a washing machine using a gentle cycle but without fabric softener or bleach. (Put bandages in a mesh laundry bag to prevent them from being tangled in the washer.)

- Do not wring or stretch these bandages while they are wet.

- These bandages can be air dried without exposure to either direct sunlight or heat sources.

- When hanging wet bandages to dry, fold them in half so that the weight of the water does not cause them to stretch.

- Before reuse, roll the bandages correctly. If rolled too loosely, they are difficult to apply. If rolled too tightly, they pre-stretch, loose their stretch, and require more frequent washing to restore their stretch.

- Bandages should be replaced when they no longer regain their stretch when washed.

Using A Bandage Winder

A bandage roller, also known as a bandage winder, is helpful in rolling bandages properly. These rollers are available as inexpensive plastic hand operated models or as a mechanized winder, such as the one shown in Figure 11-7. Although a mechanized winder is more expensive to purchase, it can be an excellent investment because it eases and speeds the rolling process. This is particularly important when ongoing bandaging is recommended. These aids can be found online by searching under "bandage winder."

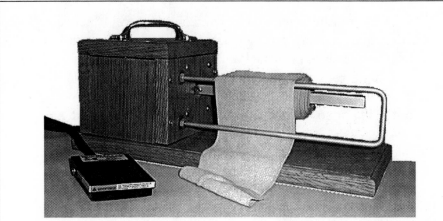

Figure 11-7: An electric bandage winder makes bandage preparation faster and easier.

Stories of Lymph Notes Members

Both of my legs are affected and I live alone. At first nightly self-bandage was like a three-ring circus act. However, I finally got the hang of it and then I started to developed carpel tunnel syndrome from the winding motions of preparing bandages. I searched for a source of an electric bandage winder. When I found one it seemed expensive; however, I've discovered that this is a great investment in taking care of myself—and I'm worth it.

Chapter 12

Home Exercise Program

Exercise is an effective way to support lymphatic system function because it increases the rate of lymph flow 15 times.[1] Exercise also helps combat the depression and fatigue associated with lymphedema while it improves your general health and well-being.

Many lymphedema treatment centers offer exercise classes. These classes are very helpful because they provide a guided exercise program plus the support of others who have lymphedema. You should exercise at home at least once a day, in addition to exercising in class.[2]

Ask your lymphedema therapist if the activities suggested here are appropriate for you. Your therapist should recommend the number of repetitions for each exercise and may suggest additional activities as part of your exercise program. Some people with lymphedema engage in vigorous sports as discussed in Chapters 13 and 16.

The exercises discussed in this chapter are specifically designed to stimulate the flow of lymph and are performed while wearing bandages or a compression garment on the affected limb.

The Exercise Setting

These quiet exercises allow you to relax as you gently move your body. They can be performed while lying comfortably on the floor, an exercise mat, or a

> **Important!**
>
> ☐ Never begin a new exercise program without first checking with your lymphedema therapist and/or your healthcare provider.
>
> ☐ Always wear your compression garment or bandages while exercising.

firm bed. Closing your eyes and listening to soothing background music as you exercise will increase your relaxation and enhance your ability to concentrate on the pleasant sensations of the muscle movements.

Deep Breathing

Deep breathing, also known as *abdominal* or *diaphragmatic breathing*, plays an important role in stimulating the flow of lymph upward through the abdomen and chest. It is also relaxing and should be performed throughout your exercise session.[3] The hand placement described here will help you learn how this breathing pattern feels:

*   Place your hands lightly on your abdomen (Figure 12-1). As you slowly breathe in, feel your hands rise as your abdomen expands. Inhaling brings fresh air into your lungs and sends oxygen flowing to all parts of your body.

*   As you slowly breathe out, feel your hands move down as your abdomen flattens. Exhaling forces stale air and waste products out of the lungs and creates space to bring in the next breath of fresh air.

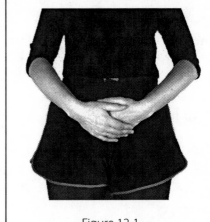

Figure 12-1

When Do You Use Deep Breathing?

☐ Your **daily routine** should include deep breathing. This can be performed anywhere at any time while you are sitting, standing, or lying down.

☐ **Start your day** with a series of deep breaths before you get out of bed to stimulate the lymphatic system, which has slowed during the night.

☐ **Self-massage** should include deep breathing before, during, and after the massage.

☐ **When you want to relax,** use deep breathing.

☐ **As you are going to sleep,** breathe deeply and relax. This also gives your lymphatic system a little boost before it slows down for the night.

Exercise Preparation and Sequence

These exercises follow a sequence of steps that enhance the flow of lymph, just like manual lymph drainage and self-massage. When you ask your therapist about what best exercises are best for you, also ask what sequence is best for you.

• Wear loose clothing so that you can move easily.

• Get into a comfortable position.

• As you slowly begin your deep breathing, take several minutes to quiet your mind so that you can concentrate on enjoying your exercises.

• Continue this relaxed deep breathing pattern throughout your exercise session.

Precautions for Exercising Under Compression

- Always exercise the unaffected side of the body first.[4] This promotes the flow of lymph within this area and prepares it to receive lymph from the affected side.

- Do not exercise to the point of exhaustion. Start with brief sessions and gradually increase your exercise time as your tolerance permits.

- Avoid exercising in a hot and humid setting.

- Stop immediately if you feel dizzy, short of breath, or uncomfortable.

- Avoid violent or strenuous movements and movements that cause pain.

General Body Movements

These exercises are performed first as a "warm up" and to prepare the lymphatics to receive the lymph that will be flowing from the limbs. Each movement is performed 10 to 20 times, unless your therapist has instructed you otherwise.

Head and Neck Movements

Gentle neck movements stimulate the terminus and prepare the lymphatic system to receive and transport the additional lymph that will be moved as you exercise.

These activities are best performed in a seated position.

- Slowly and gently, bend your neck from side to side as shown in Figure 12-2.

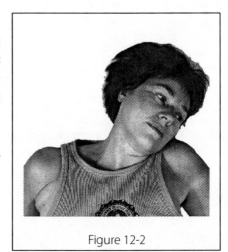

Figure 12-2

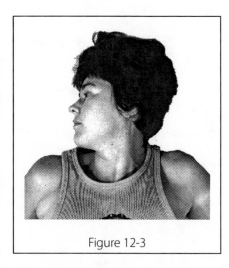

Figure 12-3

- Slowly and gently, move your head from front to back with a chin down and then chin up motion.

- Slowly and gently, rotate your head but do not force your neck beyond its comfort range (Figure 12-3).

Trunk Rotation

Trunk rotation stimulates the flow of lymph from the legs as it moves upward through the lower trunk and the chest.

- Lie flat on your back with your legs extended straight and your arms outstretched.

- Keep your right leg straight on the floor. Bend your left leg up and gently rotate it across the right leg until the left knee touches the floor. Slowly and gradually, return the left leg to its starting position lying straight and flat on the floor (Figure 12-4).

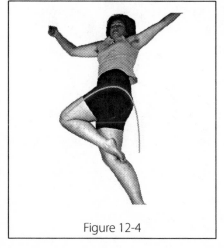

Figure 12-4

- Keep your left leg straight on the floor. Bend your right leg up and gently rotate it across the left leg until the right knee touches the floor. Slowly and gradually, return the right leg to its starting position lying straight and flat on the floor.

- Slide the right arm along the floor until it is straight above your head. Gently rotate your upper body to the left. During this movement, try to keep the backs of your knees in contact with the floor. Slowly return to lying flat on your back and gradually bring the right arm back to the side of your body.

- Slide the left arm along the floor until it is straight above your head. Gently rotate your upper body to the right. During this movement, try to keep the backs of your knees in contact with the floor. Slowly return to lying flat on your back and gradually bring the left arm back to the side of your body.

Hip Rotation

Hip rotation stimulates the flow of lymph from the legs as it moves upward through the lower trunk and the chest.

- Lie flat on your back with your legs extended straight and your arms outstretched.

- Slightly bend your knees and gently rotate your hips from side to side.

- Straighten your legs. Then bend your right knee, grasp it with your hands, and pull it straight up towards your chest. Release and gently straighten your leg.

- Bend your left knee, grasp it with your hands, and pull it up towards your chest. Release and gently straighten your leg.

Arm Exercises

The exercises are designed for those with an affected arm and can be performed while sitting or standing. Continue slow, deep breathing during these exercises.

Shoulder Exercises

- Repeat the neck rotation movements.

- Gently roll your shoulders forward and then rotate them toward the back. Return to the starting position.

- Gently bring both arms up away from your sides and gradually bring them down again, as if you were making a snow-angel.

Elbow, Wrist, and Finger Exercises

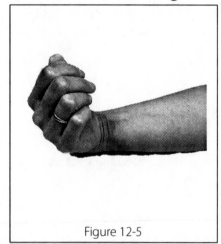

Figure 12-5

- With your arms at your sides, bring the lower portion of each arm forward by bending at the elbow. Then straighten the elbows and return the arms to your sides.

- With your arms bent at the elbows and the palms of your hands facing upward, gently bend your hands backward and then forward as far as comfortable (Figure 12-5).

- With your arms bent at the elbows and the palms of your hands facing upward, extend your fingers and gently rotate your wrists.

- With your arms bent at the elbows and the palms of your hands facing upward, extend your fingers. Bend and straighten your fingers and then move them in a rotating motion (Figure 12-6).

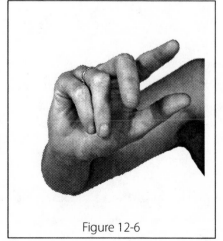

Figure 12-6

Wrist, Elbow, and Shoulder Exercises

After the finger exercises, work your way back up the arm by repeating the wrist, elbow, and shoulder motions.

Leg Exercises

These exercises are designed for those with an affected leg and are performed while standing with a sturdy chair nearby to help maintain your balance. If necessary, these exercises can be performed while seated.

Continue slow, deep breathing while performing these exercises. If both legs are affected, ask your therapist which leg exercises would be best for you.

Hip Exercises

- March in place with emphasis on the hip motion.

- While stabilizing your balance, swing your unaffected leg backward and forward. Return to a standing position.

- While stabilizing your balance, swing your affected leg backward and forward. Return to a standing position.

- While stabilizing your balance, swing your unaffected leg out toward the side. Return to a standing position.

- While stabilizing your balance, swing your affected leg out toward the side. Return to a standing position.

Knee and Ankle Exercises

- Repeat marching in place with the emphasis on bringing the knees up as high as possible.

- While stabilizing your balance, raise your unaffected leg. Bend and straighten the knee five times with the leg raised and then lower the leg to the floor.

- Repeat the previous exercise using your affected leg.

- Raise the unaffected foot off of the floor and rotate the ankle in clockwise circles. Repeat this activity, making counter-clockwise circles.

- Raise the affected foot off of the floor and rotate the ankle in clockwise circles. Repeat this activity, making counter-clockwise circles.

Foot Exercises

- Foot exercises are best performed while seated or lying down.

- Alternately bend and straighten the affected foot and unaffected foot (Figure 12-7).

- Stretch the toes of the unaffected foot upward and then downward. Move the toes apart as far as possible and wiggle them.

- Stretch the toes of the affected foot upward and then downward. Move the toes apart as far as possible and wiggle them.

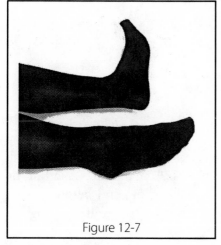

Figure 12-7

Ankle, Knee, and Hip Exercises

Work your way back up the leg in the reverse sequence:

- Raise the affected foot and bend it upward and then downward.

- Raise the unaffected foot and bend it upward and then downward.

- Raise the affected foot off of the floor and rotate the ankle in clockwise circles. Repeat this activity, making counter-clockwise circles.

- Raise the unaffected foot off of the floor and rotate the ankle in clockwise circles. Repeat this activity, making counter-clockwise circles.

- While stabilizing your balance, repeatedly bend and straighten the knee of the affected leg.

- While stabilizing your balance, repeatedly bend and straighten the knee of the unaffected leg.

- Repeat marching in place with the emphasis on bringing the knees up as high as possible.

Cool Down

After completing these exercises, relax for a few minutes while continuing your deep breathing. Complete this exercise session with another self-massage (see Chapter 10).

More Active Exercises

In addition to the exercises described above, it is equally important that you engage in more active exercise on a regular basis. Active exercises aid in the flow of lymph, weight control, a feeling of well-being, and better general health. One example of active exercise is the progressive walking program described on the next page.

Aquatic exercises are discussed in Chapter 13 and activities like hiking, scuba diving, and dragon boat racing are discussed in Chapter 16.

Walking Toward Better Health

The program presented here is a 13-week plan to help you manage your lymphedema and to improve your physical fitness in less than 40 minutes per day. When you complete this program, you will be strong enough to enjoy a one-hour walk at least three times a week.

This program involves walking at a normal pace and power walking. *Power walking* is walking at a faster than normal pace with the elbows bent while swinging the arms back and forth. You do not need weights or special equipment. You should have a pair of comfortable shoes that provide adequate support (see Chapter 9). You may want a watch or a kitchen timer to keep track of the time.

Pick a convenient place to walk that is safe and reasonably flat. Many people enjoy walking in shopping malls and large public buildings, especially early in the morning. Others prefer walking in the fresh air.

The charts beginning on the next page will help you track your progress. Each day perform the activities listed with a check box for that day. After your walk, check off your progress for the day. At the end of the week note the date that you completed this level of accomplishment.

Note: If you want to reserve one day each week to rest, that is fine. If the pace is moving ahead too rapidly for you, repeat a week as necessary, and extend the length of the program.

Walking Program—weeks 1 to 6								
Week	**S**	**M**	**T**	**W**	**T**	**F**	**S**	**Activity**
1	☐	☐	☐	☐	☐	☐	☐	Walk 5, rest 1, walk 5 minutes
2	☐		☐		☐			Walk 3, rest 1, walk 3, rest 1, walk 3, rest 1, walk 3
		☐		☐		☐	☐	Walk 5, rest 1, walk 5 minutes
3	☐		☐		☐			Walk 4, rest 1, walk 4, rest 1, walk 4, rest 1, walk 4
		☐		☐		☐	☐	Walk 6, rest 2, walk 6 minutes
4	☐		☐		☐			Walk 5, rest 1, walk 5, rest 1, walk 5, rest 1, walk 5
		☐		☐		☐	☐	Walk 7, rest 2, walk 7 minutes
5	☐		☐		☐			Walk 8, rest 2, walk 8 minutes
		☐		☐		☐	☐	Walk 6, power walk 3, walk 6 minutes
6	☐		☐		☐			Walk 10, rest 3, walk 10 minutes
		☐		☐		☐	☐	Walk 6, power walk 3, walk 6 minutes

Walking Program—weeks 7 to 13

Week	S	M	T	W	T	F	S	Activity
7	☐		☐		☐			Walk 7, power walk 3, walk 7 minutes
		☐		☐		☐	☐	Walk 5, rest 1, walk 5, rest 1, walk 5, rest 1, walk 5
8	☐		☐		☐			Walk 7, power walk 3, walk 7 minutes
		☐		☐		☐	☐	Walk 5, rest 1, walk 5, rest 1, walk 5, rest 1, walk 5
9	☐		☐		☐			Walk 10, rest 2, walk 10 minutes
		☐		☐		☐	☐	Walk 6, rest 1, walk 6, rest 1, walk 6, rest 1, walk 6
10	☐		☐		☐			Walk 10, rest 2, walk 10 minutes
		☐		☐		☐	☐	Walk 6, rest 1, walk 6, rest 1, walk 6, rest 1, walk 6
11	☐		☐		☐			Walk 12, rest 3, walk 12 minutes
		☐		☐		☐	☐	Walk 7, rest 1, walk 7, rest 1, walk 7, rest 1, walk 7
12	☐		☐		☐			Walk 15, rest 3, walk 15 minutes
		☐		☐		☐	☐	Walk 9, rest 1, walk 9, rest 1, walk 9, rest 1, walk 9
13	☐	☐	☐	☐	☐	☐	☐	Walk 30 minutes every day

Congratulations!

When you have come this far in the program, you are fit enough to enjoy a one-hour hike three times a week over different terrain.

Stories of Lymph Notes Members

A favorite part of my journey to our lymphedema support group meeting is passing a park where a Tai Chi group meets. Their movements are smooth and gentle and they look very peaceful. According to a man on the bus, who seemed to know what he was talking about, *"Tai Chi brings a wide range of health benefits to the muscular, skeletal, and circulatory systems.— and the flowing movements serve as a moving meditation that reduces stress and provides a way to cultivate body and mind."*

During refreshment time (my favorite part of the meeting), I mentioned the Tai Chi group and my interest in exploring this activity. Lorraine said she had enjoyed Tai Chi lessons— particularly performing the movements with the strange names such as *"brushing the swallow's tail."* Several of us agreed to start a Tai Chi exercise group specifically for those with lymphedema. We adopted the name of "Oh Swell Tai Chi" (and if you think this name is bad, you should have heard the suggestions we turned down).

Our Tai Chi group is now in its second year and we continue to enjoy it. We are all still active in our support group because important things happen there. We meet others who are facing the same problems we are facing or have faced. We talk, we learn from the speakers, and we encourage each other. One of my favorite changes is the increasing emphasis on the things that we can do instead of those activities that 'one with lymphedema, or at risk for it, should not attempt.'

Chapter **13**

Aquatic Therapy

The Benefits of Aquatic Therapy

Aquatic therapy, or *hydrotherapy*, exercises are performed while immersed in water.[1] These activities are beneficial for those with lymphedema for many reasons.

- The support of the water makes possible motions that could not be achieved in other settings.

- The buoyancy of the water allows exercise without heavy jarring or impact on the joints.

- Water relaxes muscles, decreases pain, and increases the sense of well-being.

- Water supplies resistance to movement that strengthens muscles and improves cardiac and respiratory conditioning.

Aquatic Therapy Precautions

Follow these basic precautions at all times:

- **Check first** with your lymphedema therapist and healthcare provider to determine if aquatic therapy is safe for you.

- **If you can't swim,** use the pool only under supervision, stay in shallow water, and wear a flotation device.

- **Stay hydrated.** Your body loses water while you are exercising in the pool. Keep a plastic water bottle handy at the side of the pool and take refreshing sips as needed. Being *hydrated* means having adequate fluids in the body.

- **Protect your affected limb.** Being immersed in water will dry the tissues of your affected limb. It is important that you apply a protective lotion over that area before going into the water. If you are going to be in the sun, use a combination of moisturizing lotion and sunscreen.

- **Use good pool hygiene.** To avoid infections, such as athlete's foot, always wear footwear when walking to and from the pool and in the shower area. After your water session, dry the skin carefully and apply an antifungal ointment or powder.

- **Protect sensitive feet.** If the soles of your feet are affected and tender, wear "pool shoes" while in the water.

Do You Need Your Compression Garment?

The hydrostatic pressure of the water against the legs is similar to that of therapeutic compression stockings. For this reason, compression stockings are not usually worn during aquatic exercises. (*Hydrostatic pressure* is the pressure exerted by water due to the weight of the column of water above it.)

Some therapists recommend wearing a compression sleeve during aquatic exercises because arms are out of the water much of the time and therefore are not subjected to hydrostatic pressure. Other therapists suggest standing immersed in the water to shoulder level instead of wearing a compression sleeve.

Your decision should be made on the recommendation of your therapist. Chlorine damages compression garments. Therefore, if you need to wear a sleeve in the water, you may want to use an old one. Also remember to bring a dry sleeve to wear when you get dressed!

Water Temperatures

Gentle exercises, such as those described in this chapter, are usually done in water that is 94° F (34° C) or slightly less.[2] Water at, or just below, this temperature feels comfortably warm and helps to relax muscles.

Strenuous exercises, such as racing or swimming laps, should be performed in much cooler water, usually between 68° F (20° C) and 86° F (30° C). For more information, see the section on "Swimming" in this chapter.

Avoid hot water that exceeds 94° F (34° C). Heat makes lymphedema worse and being in very warm water can cause complications because it raises the core temperature of the body.

Hot Tub Caution

Soaking in a hot tub sounds great. Unfortunately, the heat increases the danger of swelling for those with, or at risk of developing, lymphedema.[3]

- If your leg is potentially affected by lymphedema, a hot tub should be avoided

- If your arm is potentially affected by lymphedema, you could try a *brief* soak in a hot tub if you keep the affected arm out of the water. Pay close attention. When you begin to feel warm, get out of the hot tub. As you dry off, drink lots of water to replenish the fluids you lost while in the tub.

Jacuzzis

The bubbling action of warm, *not hot*, water in a Jacuzzi can be beneficial. When the pattern of the air jets is set with a slight pause between bursts of bubbles it mimics the gentle stroking motion of manual lymph drainage. These bubbles are particularly beneficial in the neck area where they relax the muscles and stimulate the lymph nodes in the neck and at the base of the skull.

Seawater

Seawater is a beneficial medium for aquatic therapy because it supports the body and it also kills many bacteria on the skin. A saltwater pool is an excellent setting for aquatic exercises and therapy sessions in a controlled environment. Seawater, enjoyed in its natural setting, is also a wonderful way to relax, have fun, enjoy the benefits of saltwater, and exercise.

Seawater Precautions

- If you have lymphedema of the lower extremities, always wear protective footwear when walking on the beach or exercising in the water.

- Before using a saltwater pool, apply a lubricating lotion to prevent drying out of the affected limb.

- When enjoying seawater outside, always wear a good lubricating lotion and sunscreen and reapply as necessary.

Exercising in the Water

Some lymphedema treatment centers offer aquatic or water aerobic classes. If your center does not provide this service, ask your therapist for information about water exercises that you can perform on your own. Included in this chapter are frequently recommended aquatic exercises. Before trying them, ask your therapist if they are appropriate for you. Your therapist may recommend additional aquatic exercises that are specific to your needs.

Start slow. If you have never performed water exercises before, it is wise to start with short sessions and build it up to fifty or sixty minutes. Because water changes the dynamics and sensitivity of the body, an aquatic exercise session should not last longer than one hour.

Be creative. The exercises included here are not an exhaustive list. In addition to those exercises suggested by your therapist, you may want to add other exercises. When changing an exercise program, always make changes slowly.

Lymphedema-affected tissues tend to have a delayed response, so a problem may not appear immediately. Therefore it is advisable to try only a few repetitions of a new exercise in a single session. If you do not develop any negative reaction, such as pain or extreme fatigue, try a few more repetitions at your next pool session.

Walking in the Water

Walking in the water is an excellent warm-up activity to start your pool session. The more relaxed you are, and the slower you walk, the better it is for your lymphatic system. The recommended time for this activity ranges from three to ten minutes of gentle walking. As you walk in chest level water, concentrate on deep breathing as described in Chapter 11 and walk properly by:

- Place your heel on the pool floor and roll on the outer edge of the sole of your foot toward the ball of the foot.

- Lift your heel and push off with the toes and bring the foot forward.

- Place the heel of the other foot on the pool floor and roll on the outer edge of the sole toward the ball of the foot. Lift the heel and push toes off to take a step forward and land on the other heel.

This basic step can be alternated with walking backward to improve stability of the spine and strengthen the back muscles, or walking sideways to improve stability of the pelvis and hips.

By using a variety of walking exercises the muscle pumps are activated and can aid in improving lymph drainage.

An impact-free alternative to this activity is to wear a flotation belt and "walk" in deeper water.

Arm Movements While Walking

These movements can be varied as you continue to enjoy walking:

- Let your arms trail behind you and enjoy the sensation of the water flowing over them.

- If your arm is affected, let your arms float in front of you as you walk, and gently move them from side-to-side on the surface of the water.

- After your initial warm-up period, increase your pace and swing your arms as if you were power walking. During power walking the elbows are bent while swinging your arms back and forth. As your arms swing forward, bring them up toward the surface of the water. Power walking is explained in Chapter 12.

Relaxing Shoulder Rolls

Stand in water up to your shoulders, breathe deeply, and relax.

- Let your arms float on the water in front of you.

- Roll your shoulders upward, backward, downward, and forward. Your extended, but relaxed, arms will passively follow these movements.

- Repeat these movements in reverse rotation.

Head Movements

Stand in water up to your shoulders, breathe deeply, and relax.

- **Head Tilt.** Slowly tilt your head from the center to one side, then to the other side, and return your head to the center.

- **Head Turn.** Turn your head to one side and then to the center, then to the other side and back to the center again.

- **Shoulder Roll and Head Turn.** Relax and repeat head movements with the shoulder rolls.

Hand Pressing

Stand in water deep enough for your arms to move comfortably on the surface of the water. Press the palms of your hands together on the surface of the water and release. This movement, which increases lymph drainage from the arms and shoulders, should be repeated several times.

Knee Bouncing in the Water

In water that is between chest and shoulder deep, stand straight with your back supported flat against the side of the pool.

- Bounce one knee towards your chest and return that foot to the floor.

- Repeat these movements with the other leg.

Floater Activities

A floater, such as a ball or a plastic foam noodle, is an excellent exercise aid for use in a pool facility.

Pushing a floater down. As you breathe in, hold the floater in front of you and push it down until your arms are fully extended. While breathing out, and with your arms still fully extended, slowly let the floater come back up to the surface.

Sitting on a noodle. Sit on a noodle as if you are sitting on a swing. Bring both knees upward toward the chest and then push them outward again. This improves deep breathing, supports drainage of the inguinal nodes, and improves your balance.

Standing on a noodle. Begin by sitting on the noodle. Bring your feet up and move into a squatting position on the noodle. Use your feet to push the noodle down to the pool floor and stand on the noodle. This activity improves abdominal breathing, supports drainage of the groin nodes, and improves your balance and flexibility. *Caution:* You could lose your balance while learning to do this. Do not try this if you have balance or mobility issues. Select a location that is not too close to the edge of the pool or near other swimmers.

Walking on the noodle. Once standing on the noodle, take small steps from one side to the other side of the noodle. To maintain your balance, you may need to turn your feet as you move. This activity improves your balance and muscle strength and flexibility. The movement stimulates the lymphatic pumps in your legs and feet (see Section IV). *Caution:* You could lose your balance while learning to do this. Do not try this if you have balance or mobility issues. Select a location that is not too close to the edge of the pool or near other swimmers while practicing.

Swimming

Swimming is an all-in-one exercise that encourages deep breathing, improves muscle tone, and increases kidney and heart functions. Swimming also stimulates the lymphatic system and increases your sense of well-being.

- The **breaststroke** is recommended for either an affected arm or leg because it involves gentle stretching motions of arms and legs.

- The **butterfly stroke** is not recommended for an affected arm because it requires strenuous repetitive movements.

- **Racing and swimming laps** should only be undertaken after consultation with your therapist. The decision depends on your condition and your training. If you enjoyed these activities before you had lymphedema, return to them slowly. Allow time to determine how your body reacts and build up your endurance slowly.

Snow Angels in the Water

Making "snow angels" in the pool is another excellent exercise. This activity requires floating and if this is a problem for you, a flotation aid may be needed. Also, you need space in the pool to move through the water.

- Float on your back, with your arms at your sides and your legs extended. Slide your arms upward across the surface of the water until your arms are extended above your head with your hands touching.

- At the same time, move your legs outward across the surface of the water toward the side.

- Move your arms and legs downward at the same time -- as if you were making a snow angel in the water. This motion will propel you through the water.

Repeat several times being careful not to bump into others or the side of the pool.

Self-Massage

Complete your aquatic exercise session by performing self-massage again. This will help to continue moving the lymph flow that has been stimulated by the activities and motion of the water against the body. It also helps to reduce delayed onset muscle fatigue from your exercise session.

Stories of Lymph Notes Members

Summers and sandy beaches are my favorite memories. When I was little we lived in Florida, so playing in the sand and swimming in the gulf were part of our everyday life. Now that I'm married and have a family, our tradition is to have at least one beach vacation each year!

Two years ago all of that changed when I was diagnosed with ovarian cancer. Survival became my number one priority. As treatment progressed, and survival looked more promising, growing back my hair, which I had always worn long, moved up the priority list. Finally my treatments were complete, I had a new short hairdo, and I was looking forward to getting back to the beach with my family.

Before we were able to get there, I developed lymphedema in both legs! Walking was difficult, my legs looked terrible, and those bandages will never make a fashion statement! But my story has a happy ending.

With excellent treatment things have gotten better. My mobility has improved and I've progressed to compression hose for daytime wear. Better yet, my therapist assures me that the long walks on the beach are excellent exercise and swimming in the salt water is recommended for those with lymphedema.

So we are headed back on the beach again! Look for me. I'll be the one making the fashion statement with a sarong to cover the compression hose -- or you may find that sarong casually dropped on the sand as I go splashing into the healing saltwater!

Chapter **14**

Nutrition Tips

While there is no special diet that will prevent or treat lymphedema, it has been determined that good nutrition is an essential part of managing the stress that lymphedema places on the body. *Good nutrition* is defined as a well-balanced food intake that contains all of the essential nutrients in the proper quantities while enabling you to maintain your appropriate weight.

Maintaining your appropriate weight is a key phrase here. For those with lymphedema, being overweight makes the condition worse and more difficult to treat. For those at risk for lymphedema, the more excess weight you carry, the greater the potential for developing lymphedema. In addition, excess weight increases the risk of complications as discussed in Chapter 6.

Evaluating Your Weight

According to the Centers for Disease Control and Prevention (CDC), the Body Mass Index (BMI) is a useful tool for evaluating the weight of adults over 20 years of age. This calculation based on height and weight, is one of the measures used to evaluate the risks associated with excess weight.

Look up your BMI online (see www.nhlbisupport.com/bmi), ask your doctor, or calculate it yourself:

• In pounds and inches, BMI is: (weight*703)/(height*height).

- In kilograms and meters, BMI is: weight/(height*height).

Obesity and Morbid Obesity

In adults, *obesity* is defined as a BMI greater than 30. *Morbid obesity* is defined as a BMI greater than 39, or being more than 100 pounds over the established weight standards for your height, age, and sex.

Weight at these levels is classified as a disease and often causes other serious conditions including diabetes, heart disease, high blood pressure, stroke, and lymphedema. For more details, see "How Fat Affects the Flow of Lymph" in Section IV.

Once you have identified your healthy weight, reaching and maintaining this goal depends on establishing and following a successful weight control program. This program needs to be one that works for you and can be an ongoing lifestyle change. You may prefer an organized program with a support group.

This program should include the following elements:

- A **holistic approach** that combines proper nutrition, exercise, knowing why you overeat, and understanding how to make the appropriate changes.

- **Awareness** of what you eat, when you eat, and how much you eat (portion size, number of portions). Try keeping a food diary for a week and recording everything you eat; you may be surprised how much you eat.

- A **well-balanced diet** that includes all food groups in moderation so that excess calories are not consumed. Begin by making one or two dietary changes that you can maintain; then make more changes when you are ready.

- **Eat more fruits, vegetables, and whole grain products** that are nutritious and filling, yet have few calories per serving.

- **Eat fewer sugary foods,** such as cookies and candy, which supply fat and empty calories with almost no nutritional value.

- **Drink fewer sugary beverages,** such as soft drinks, that supply empty calories with little or no nutritional value. Drink water instead.

- **Eat fewer processed foods** that are high in fats, sodium, and calories but have a low nutrient content.

- **Exercise** to help achieve and maintain your ideal weight by increasing your metabolism, improving muscle tone, and enhancing your sense of well-being. Exercise and improved muscle tone also increase the effectiveness of compression in the treatment of lymphedema.

- **Set achievable goals!** Don't plan your entire weight loss as a single goal. Set an achievable goal such as a 10 pound weight loss over 10 weeks. Celebrate your success and move on to the next 10 pound loss.

- **Evaluate setbacks in a positive light.** These are not failures. They are a sign that it is time to review your weight control plan and goals to determine if changes need to be made.

Chemotherapy Weight Gain

A weight gain of as much as 15 pounds is frequently associated with chemotherapy. The causes are not clear, it is assumed to be due to slowed metabolism and a lack of physical activity. If you are beginning chemotherapy, request a consultation with a nutritionist who can help you have ample nutrition and minimize weight gain.

Weight Fluctuations

It is normal for weight to fluctuate slightly from day-to-day and at different times during the day. For this reason, most weight loss programs usually recommend weighing yourself only once a week and always weighing at the same time of day.

If you have lymphedema, your weight will increase as swelling increases and decrease as swelling is reduced. Lymphatic fluid is heavier than normal body tissues and about the same density as water, 8 pounds per gallon or 1 kilogram per liter.

Despite these fluctuations, it is still recommended that you set a target desirable weight range and move toward this goal without worrying about these temporary lymphedema-related gains and losses.

Vitamins, Minerals, and Supplements

Research has established that coping with chronic stress depletes the body's supply of vitamins, minerals, and other nutrients. An adequate daily intake of nutrients is important for maintaining health in the presence of stress.

Some dietitians maintain that all necessary vitamins, minerals, and other nutrients can be obtained through a well-balanced diet; others recommend specific supplements. A consultation with a qualified professional dietitian or nutritionist can be very helpful in making the right supplement decisions to meet your needs.

Dietary Proteins and Lymphedema

Because lymphedema is associated with the presence of protein-rich lymph, the question often arises, *"Should I stop eating protein so there won't be protein in this fluid?"* The answer to this question is, *"No! Do not stop eating protein. It won't solve your problem."* In fact, a shortage of protein, or the inability to digest protein, can cause swelling.

This emphatic answer is easier to understand when you understand the differences between dietary proteins and the high-protein fluid associated with lymphedema.

Dietary Proteins

Dietary proteins are found in many of the foods we eat. Meat, fish, dairy products, soy, beans, and eggs are examples of high protein foods.

Proteins are important for good health because:

- Proteins are the building blocks of the body.

- Proteins are the only nutrients that can repair worn-out tissues and build new ones.

- Proteins are used by the body to manufacture essential hormones.

- Proteins have a role in building antibodies to fight infections.

- Proteins aid the blood in transporting oxygen and nutrients.

- Proteins are essential to the clotting of blood.

The goal for each individual should be to eat the appropriate amount of dietary protein to meet their nutritional needs. For a person who is eating 2,000 calories per day, the recommended daily value is 50 grams of protein. This protein should come from a variety of sources, not only meat, and include only a minimum amount of fat.

When There is a Shortage of Dietary Proteins

When there are not enough dietary proteins available to meet the needs of the body, proteins are taken from the tissues and muscles to maintain the proper protein level of the blood. A severe shortage of dietary proteins will weaken connective tissues and causes them to swell. This is known as *hunger edema* and it can be seen in the swollen bellies of starving children.

Seriously restricting the intake of dietary protein in an effort to control the swelling of lymphedema does not help. It has just the opposite effect: It increases the amount of swelling that is present. It also weakens the muscles and other tissues.

A Low Sodium Diet is Not Indicated

High salt intake can contribute to hypertension and certain types of edema associated with cardiac conditions. However, the swelling of lymphedema is not related to excess salt intake. Although a low sodium diet may be recommended to reduce fluid retention due to other causes, a low sodium diet is not an effective treatment for lymphedema.

The Importance of Being Well Hydrated

The term *hydrated* describes the state of having adequate fluids in the body and maintaining this balance is an essential part of good health. The generally accepted guidelines are to drink at least six to eight 8-ounce glasses of fluid a day. This fluid intake can be in the form of juice, milk, soup, or other beverages; however, it should include at least two glasses of water.

Drinking adequate fluids to keep the body properly hydrated is extremely important for those with lymphedema. Reducing fluid intake in an attempt to reduce the swelling of lymphedema doesn't work. Instead of having the desired effect, reduced fluid intake causes the protein-rich lymph to attract fluid from the other parts of the body, thus increasing the swelling in the affected area.

Staying well hydrated by drinking plenty of water is especially important after an MLD or pump treatment to flush out the fluids that were moved during treatment.

Tips for Staying Hydrated

☐ Drink more in hot weather and in dry conditions when the body loses fluids more rapidly due to perspiration.

☐ Water, milk, and fruit juices are excellent fluid sources.

☐ Always carry a water bottle. Partially freezing the bottle will help to keep the water cool in hot weather.

☐ Sip from your water bottle at least once every hour. Drink more often if you are thirsty.

☐ Caffeinated drinks including coffee, tea, chocolate, soft drinks, and some alcoholic beverages should be consumed in moderation. *Caffeine* is a mild diuretic and reduces the level of body fluids by encouraging the kidneys to excrete more urine.

Stories of Lymph Notes Members

I am a lymphedema therapist, and I am also doing the Atkins Diet. Since my patients frequently as about diet, I'd like to share my thoughts regarding the Atkins Diet and lymphedema.

Most people who have lymphedema have learned that the fluid that comprises the edema is a combination of water and protein. This naturally leads to the question "If I eat less protein, will I have less edema?" The answer is no. The dietary protein you ingest is in no way related to the protein content of the edema. It is two entirely different systems at work. Also being at your optimal weight is one of the best ways to manage lymphedema and prevent worsening.

On a personal note, I have lost 17 pounds on the Atkins Diet in about two months. The best advice I can give anyone who is interested is to pick up the Atkins book, read it all the way through, and follow the guidelines. I have seen people get into trouble with malnutrition by simply going "low carb" all of a sudden. The Atkins book gives a clear rationale for why the diet works, as well as great guidelines about choosing foods as you continue along the weight loss path.

As a therapist, I am thrilled when patients are concerned with their weight and want to take positive steps to change. I encourage them to get clearance from their physician before starting any diet (to make sure that heart, lungs, kidneys are functioning normally). It's also nice to have a before and after cholesterol, blood pressure, and resting heart rate testing to see if your diet is helping you make the changes you want.

Christine Thomas, PT, CLT-LANA

Chapter **15**

Keeping a Health Journal

A health journal isn't just a record of aches, pains, and pills. It is an organized approach to managing your lymphedema care by gathering all of the lymphedema-related information in a ring binder. This creates a convenient resource for your use, a valuable reference during medical visits, a systematic method of evaluating your progress, and a system for managing information you may need to appeal an insurance denial.

Create Your Health Journal

A ring binder is suggested because it can easily be divided into sections and pages can be added or removed as necessary. Also, since most ring binders have pockets, this is a good place to keep the information brochures you receive. A spiral bound notebook can also work for this purpose, some come with section dividers.

Organize Your Records into Sections

Organize your records in a way that makes it easy for you to keep them up-to-date. The sections and their sequence depends on what works best for you. Section headings might include:

• Calendar

- Visit records

- Current medications

- Healthcare team roster

- Medical history

- Lymphedema records

- Compression garment records

- Hospitalization records

Calendar

A calendar, preferably by month, makes a great place to record dates of appointments, treatments, or developments such as infections. If you have one month per sheet, organize the sheets so that the current month is on top. Keeping the pages from past months creates an easily accessed record of important dates, such as when you received chemotherapy. Make notes, or put sticky notes on future pages to remind you about things that you need to follow-up.

Visit Records

You can improve the level of communication and the effectiveness of your healthcare visits by taking a few minutes to organize your thoughts and questions before your appointment. Make a page for each visit that includes:

- Your name, the date, and healthcare provider.

- Reasons for this visit, including any changes that have occurred since the last visit.

- A list of the questions you would like to have answered and space to record the answers; consider making a copy of your question list to give to your healthcare provider. If you don't understand the answer to your question, ask for clarification.

After the visit, store the sheet in your ring binder with the most recent one on top.

Current Medications

At the end of each visit, update the list of medications you are taking so that you'll have accurate information the next time you are asked. Having a written list makes it easier for a provider to spot potential drug interactions and avoids confusion due to similar sounding names.

- **Head the list with your name and the date it was updated.**

- **If you have any allergies,** particularly to medications, note these on your list.

- **Note the name and telephone number of your pharmacy.** This makes a ready reference for the question, "What is the phone number of the pharmacy you use?"

- **List each medication separately.** For each prescription note the following information: the name of the drug, the dose per pill and per day, what condition this medication is being administered to treat, and the name of the prescribing doctor.

- **List over-the-counter medications** such as aspirin, antihistamines, antacids, vitamins, and herbal or other supplements. Your physician needs this information because some of these medications can interact with prescription medications.

In addition to having this information in your health journal, it is also a good idea to carry a copy of your list of current medications in your purse or wallet. You never know when you might need it.

Also use this section to record the information that you need to refill your prescriptions. Your calendar is a good place to note the date when each prescription is due to be refilled.

Either at the back of this section, or in a separate section, you may want to store the "Patient Information Sheets" that you receive with your prescriptions.

Healthcare Team Roster

Many patients with lymphedema see multiple healthcare providers for different specialties. The roster lists the contact information for each provider in one place.

- **List each healthcare provider who is currently or has recently treated you.** Include each provider's name, specialty, telephone, and fax numbers. Including an address is optional.

- **If a physician is no longer treating you,** note the beginning and ending dates of the care provided. For example, if you have completed radiation therapy, list the name of your radiologist and note the beginning and final dates of treatment.

- **List your lymphedema therapist's** name, telephone, and fax numbers.

Medical History

Write down the answers to those frequently asked questions about major illnesses, surgeries (with dates), and family history. This will make it faster and easier for you to give an accurate history.

- If you are presently under treatment for cancer, note the dates of the treatments and what has been done to date.

- If you have completed cancer treatment, summarize this treatment by noting the date of diagnosis plus the dates (beginning and ending) of the different types of treatment.

Lymphedema Records

Lymphedema is a chronic condition that is not going away. However, your memory of the details may fade. Keeping a record helps you organize information about treatments you have received and problems you encountered. It may also prove to be very helpful in dealing with your insurance company should treatment be denied. You may want to subdivide this section by topic as explained below.

The Diagnosis of Lymphedema

Note the date and name of the physician who first diagnosed your lymphedema. Also include details about the initial treatment recommendations you received.

Note the cause of your lymphedema. This could be **primary** (inherited), **secondary** (due to the factors described in Chapter 1), or **idiopathic** (*Idiopathic* means of unknown cause).

Note the early warning signs you experienced plus the reasons and date when you finally sought a diagnosis. If other diagnoses were considered, include that information too.

Treatment Records

Note the date and name of the facility where you started treatment. Include details about treatment that was provided, such as information about your intensive. Including dates and details of individual visits is optional. If you change treatment facilities, note the ending date and reason for changing. If you don't recall these details, you can request a copy of your record from the facility.

Limb Measurements

One important way in which the progress of lymphedema treatment is tracked is by measuring the size of the lymphedema-affected limb at specific points. This process is known as *volumetrics* and your therapist will record these measurements periodically.

You can use a similar method to evaluate the effectiveness of your self-management program at home. Ask your therapist to teach you how to take measurements at about three points. Follow these instructions and carefully take these measurements once a week at home. By recording your findings you create a progressive record that indicates if the limb volume is decreasing, staying the same, or increasing in size.

Complications Record

Each time you have an infection or lymphedema-related complication that requires medical attention, note the following information:

- Date of first symptoms and the cause (if known).

- Name of treating healthcare provider and dates of treatment.

- A list of the antibiotics that were administered and your reaction to each. Note any antibiotics that were not effective.

- If you had a negative reaction to any of these medications, note it here. Then add this medicine to the allergy section on your medication list.

Compression Garment Record

Compression garments should be evaluated every six months and replaced as necessary. When you get a new garment, note the date and where you got the garment and add a reminder on your calendar to have the garment checked in six months. After your garment's checkup, schedule new reminder.

Hospitalization Records

Ideally, every hospital patient would have an able-bodied advocate, or a team of advocates, to look out for them at all times. Unfortunately this is not always practical. However, maintaining an ongoing record can improve your hospital experience.

Keeping Track

Organize a letter or legal size note pad to record the events of each day of the hospitalization. This note pad stays in the room with the patient and is used by the advocate to create a sequential record of the day's events.

- On the first page list the names and specialties of the patient's physicians. Leave space here to add more names.

- Start a fresh page for each day. Date the page and note the prescribed medications and the times they are due to be administered.

- If the patient has any known allergies to medications, note these at the top of each page as a reminder to the advocate.

- Note the time, name of the caregiver, and name of each treatment or service that is provided.

- When medications are being administered, for ask the name of each and check this against the master list at the top of the page.

- Ask the nurse on duty if medications have not been administered at the appropriate time; however, allow some flexibility for busy staff.

- When a physician visits, record his or her name and specialty. Note what was said, including information such as new tests being ordered, medication changes, or discussion about the patient's discharge.

- When the physician is changing or adding medications, ask questions such as, "How will this new medication interact with the other drugs the patient is taking?" If the patient has a drug allergy, always mention this to the prescribing physician.

- Note information about laboratory test results. You may want to request a copy of the test results. When you get the report, look for the arrows that indicate results that are abnormal, i.e. either too high or too low.

- If there is a change in the patient's condition during the day, record what happened and how it was treated.

Using This Record

Your record of the events can be a comprehensive and helpful record to the physician of what has occurred during the day. It may even provide the physician with insights that are not obvious from the patient's chart.

Chapter **16**

Having Fun

Of necessity, much of this book deals with warnings about how to live safely with lymphedema. Having fun, despite having lymphedema, is an equally important part of life. Studies have shown that laughing stimulates the immune system, improves your health, and enhances your enjoyment of life. So too does taking part in activities that you enjoy.

The Value of Common Sense

A recurring theme among these precautions is to avoid strenuous, repetitive activities. This is good advice because lymphedema-affected tissues often have a delayed reaction to stress. However, in addition to being cautious, listening to your body and using your own good common sense are equally important.

Every individual with lymphedema is unique in terms of the physical challenges they face. Some were in excellent physical shape and very active before this illness. For others, the development of lymphedema is yet another physical challenge to be overcome. Everyone should be able to find fun activities to suit his or her physical condition and tastes.

It is prudent to consult your healthcare provider or lymphedema therapist before beginning a new sport or strenuous activity.

Returning to a Favorite Sport

Lymphedema-affected muscles and joints will respond differently to sports that require strength and repetitive motions such as tennis, basketball, golf, or bowling. However, there are no iron clad rules about engaging in these activities, and decisions must be made on an individual basis. If you enjoyed these sports before you had lymphedema, and playing them again is important to you, explore the possibilities.

These basics will increase your chances of being successful in returning to your favorite sports.

1. Check with your physician or lymphedema therapist.

2. When you play, wear your compression garment.

3. Start with short and moderate sessions.

4. Stop before you become fatigued.

Monitor how your affected limb responds to these sessions. If it responds well to these shorter sessions, gradually increase your training in order to return to your former playing schedule.

Finding a New Activity: Dragon Boat Racing

A group of case studies among women treated for breast cancer has demonstrated that the advice to avoid repetitive exercise is not necessarily accurate.[1] Dragon boat racing is the activity that most dramatically proves this advice to be wrong.[2] *Dragon boat racing* is a sport in which 22 to 26 paddlers, who are working very hard, row to the beat of a drum and race in competition with other similar boats.

This colorful activity requires upper body strength and repetitive motion, yet women who are at risk for lymphedema, and many who have developed it, are enjoying this sport. They work under the guidance of qualified trainers as the team members build their skills and strength to the level at which

Stories of Lymph Notes Members

I have had lymphedema in both legs since I was 28 years old, I'm 43 now. I live with this disease every single day and I know how hard it is. Until 5 years ago my legs continued to get worse and I estimated that I was about a year away from being in a wheel chair. If you had seen my legs then, you would have never imagined I would be where I am today with them.

I refused to let this disease get me down any longer and I learned to fight back. It's been a lot of hard work. I started with MLD treatment, wore compression aids for about three years, and now all I have to wear is a mild compression stocking on each leg. My doctor and I decided to try something "different". I used to be a runner. I was told I would never run again.

Well, I am a bit stubborn. So what I did, with my doctor's permission, was to wrap my legs as tight as possible and started walking on my treadmill. Then I progressed to running. Not only did I loose weight, which I needed, but my leg improved drastically.

Now I bike, fish, walk, and run. I have most of my life back. It is not the same as it was before but it is better than after the lymphedema attacked me!

they are able to successfully take part in competition. Other benefits of this activity, in addition to building physical health, are renewed self-confidence, learning new skills, and sharing the support of teammates.

Dragon boat racing is not for everyone; however, it is an excellent example of how new opportunities and challenges are available despite having lymphedema, if you seek them out.

Travel Tips

Having lymphedema, or being at risk for it, should not stop you from traveling. You may want to modify some travel plans and incorporate these precautions:

- Wear a "Medic Alert" bracelet or necklace to make emergency medical personnel aware that you have lymphedema. This should be an everyday routine!

- Before you travel, ask your health care provider about carrying antibiotics with you as a precautionary measure in case you develop an infection.

- Before you travel, ask your healthcare provider for a "note" to carry that explains that you have lymphedema. You may need to show this to airport security if there are questions about bandages or compression garments. It also may be helpful if you have a problem and require medical treatment.

- Plan your travels at a more relaxed pace to minimize stress and to allow for extra rest as necessary.

- Wear your compression garments when traveling by plane.[3] Changes in cabin pressure, plus the added stress of travel, make maintaining a normal or increased compression schedule essential.

- If your legs are affected by lymphedema, wear your compression garment but do not remove your shoes on the plane. The changing cabin pressure will accentuate the lymphedema and may make it difficult to put your shoes on later.

- If you use a compression aid, you may want to wear it while traveling rather than having it take up a lot of suitcase space.

- Pack wisely to minimize the weight of your suitcase and carry-on. This is advisable no matter which area is affected by lymphedema, because "wrestling" with heavy luggage places a strain on the entire body!

- Carry a mini-first aid kit that includes disinfectant wipes, antibiotic cream, and band-aids.

- When enjoying outdoor activities, it is important that you wear a high SPF sunscreen under your compression garment.

- When outdoors, wear insect repellent. Long sleeves or trousers are also recommended to protect the affected limb.

- If traveling in a dry climate, take extra precautions to keep the skin of the affected limb well moisturized. In a hot and humid climate, powder is recommended to help control perspiration.

- Drink lots of water! Avoid drinking alcohol, coffee, and caffeinated soft drinks. Instead of meeting your need for water, these beverages increase the amount of fluid that the body excretes. Your best choice is to always carry a water bottle and to keep drinking from it.

Saunas and Steam Rooms

Saunas and steam rooms are designed to raise your body temperature and to make you sweat. Exposure to extreme heat can increase the swelling of lymphedema. In those at risk, it can cause secondary lymphedema to develop. Therefore, saunas and steam rooms usually should be avoided by those with or at risk for lymphedema.[4]

Scuba Diving and Snorkeling

If you enjoyed scuba diving before having lymphedema, you will probably be able to enjoy this sport again. You may find that swimming and diving are beneficial because the pressure of water has a similar effect to that of compression bandaging.[5]

Normal safety precautions taken by scuba divers should always be followed. It is also important to protect the affected limb against possible injury by wearing a full-body wet suit. If the hand is affected, wear gloves to protect against injury.

Snorkeling precautions are similar to those for enjoying seawater. If returning to this sport after having acquired lymphedema, your outings should be shorter than usual until you are certain how the lymphedema affected limb will react to this level of activity. *And don't forget the sunscreen!*

Hiking and Backpacking

If you have lymphedema affecting your leg, your condition will determine whether or not these activities are advised. If lymphedema affects your arm, you probably can enjoy these activities. You'll want to take these precautions:

- Always wear your compression garment.

- Don't forget sunscreen and insect repellent.

- Train adequately by starting with short hikes while carrying a light backpack. You may find that a fanny pack or hip pack is better for you.

- Gradually increase the distance and pack weight until you've reached the desired levels.

- Avoid outings in extremely hot, humid weather and at very high elevations.

- Rest frequently. Don't push until you are fatigued and overheated.

- Always carry a water bottle with you and use it to stay well hydrated.

- Consider using a long walking stick, carried in the affected hand. This keeps your arm supported and in an elevated position.

- Carry a first aid kit that includes an antibiotic just in case you develop signs of an infection.

Having Fun on a Trampoline

Bouncing on a trampoline for about 15 minutes a day is an excellent way to stimulate the flow of lymph because lymph moves upward through the lymphatic system with every bounce. It is also a good way to have fun and to reduce stress.

Trampoline Equipment

A small 24-inch trampoline with a full suspension system (shock absorbing legs) and a safety rail is commonly used for this purpose. It is important that you hold onto the safety rail until you are certain that you are stable on the trampoline when it is in motion.

How to Bounce

Safety is essential here and high vigorous bouncing *is not* important or recommended.

- Pay attention to how you feel and never push to the point of exhaustion, pain, or the danger of falling.

- Start low, slow, and for only a few minutes.

- Begin with a warm-up session that is no more strenuous than doing knee bends with your feet on the trampoline.

- Keeping your knees slightly bent, increase your activity to low bounces, no more than two inches off the surface.

- If you are able, very carefully increase this to higher bounces and arm motions similar to jumping jacks.

- Reverse this sequence with a warm-down of low bounces and finally just knee bends.

Wheelchair Bound Trampoline Use

Some therapists suggest "bouncing" for wheelchair-bound individuals. The patient's feet are placed on the trampoline while someone else causes it to bounce. Although the patient is passive, the lymphatic system receives the benefits of the motion that is transmitted through the legs.

Yoga

The deep breathing associated with yoga is beneficial because it stimulates the flow of lymph through the trunk. The relaxation associated with yoga is also beneficial because it aids in reducing stress. Holding a yoga posture does not provide the same lymphatic benefits as more active forms of exercise. Therefore, if you enjoy yoga, it can be an excellent part of your exercise program, but it should not replace activities that require more varied muscle movements.

Shall We Dance?

Ballroom, swing, line, Latin, Hip Hop, or other dance forms are a great way to have fun, socialize, and get excellent exercise. According to Sherry Lebed Davis, who conducts special programs for those with lymphedema, *"Increasing muscular activity in a slow, smooth, rhythmic manner, improves the flow of lymph. Also the stretch and release of the skin during these exercises opens the 'drain' and further improves this flow."* [6]

Before beginning any new form of exercise it is important to check with your healthcare provider and your lymphedema therapist.

Understanding the Lymphatic System

Two Circulatory Systems

The human body is commonly described as having one circulatory system, the **cardiovascular system**. The **lymphatic system** is described separately. In fact, the lymphatic system combined with the cardiovascular system creates a second 'circulatory' system. Each plays a different, yet complementary, role in caring for the cells of the body.[1] These systems are compared in the figures on the following pages.

Functions of the Lymphatic System

The lymphatic system has many important functions, including:

- Draining excess fluid from the *interstitial* or *intercellular spaces*, the area between the cells of tissues.

- Removing waste including debris, dead blood cells, pathogens, and toxins. *Pathogens* are disease-producing microorganisms such as bacteria and viruses. *Toxins* are harmful or poisonous substances.

- Enabling the immune system to destroy cancer cells and pathogens.

Figure IV-1: *The Cardiovascular System*

Blood is visible and damage to blood vessels is observed as bleeding or bruising.

Blood consists of liquid plasma with circulating blood cells and platelets. Average blood volume is 4-6 quarts or liters.

Blood is pumped by the heart at the rate of between 60 to 120 heartbeats per minute. This rate is measured as pulse.

Blood flows in a continuous loop throughout the body via arteries, capillaries, and veins.

Blood is responsible for distributing oxygen, nutrients, and hormones to the cells.

Blood is filtered by the kidneys.

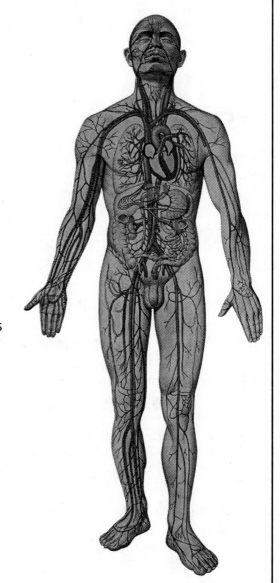

Figure IV-2: *The Lymphatic System*

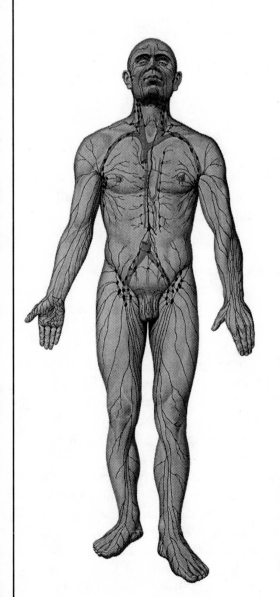

Lymph is nearly invisible and damage to the lymphatic vessels is difficult to detect.

Lymph is a clear to milky white fluid with no circulating cells of its own. Average lymph volume is 1-2 quarts or liters.

Lymph does not have a central pump. Lymphatic angions contract at the rate of 5 to 7 "beats" per minute.

Lymph flows in one direction through a closed circuit of lymphatic vessels

Lymph is responsible for collecting and removing waste products and protein molecules from the tissues.

Lymph is filtered by lymph nodes.

- Circulating lymphocytes through the lymphatic system and the blood-stream. *Lymphocytes* are white blood cells that secrete antibodies and destroy invading organisms.

- Returning protein molecules and fluid to the cardiovascular system.

- Absorbing fats and fat-soluble vitamins in the digestive system.

The Formation of Lymph

Blood plasma is a yellowish solution of ions, small molecules, and soluble proteins. Red blood cells, white blood cells, and platelets (cell fragments that initiate blood clotting) are suspended in the plasma. Each milliliter of blood contains approximately 5 billion red blood cells and 7 million white blood cells.

Plasma from the cardiovascular system flows out through the walls of the blood capillaries into the spaces between the cells. Known here as *tissue fluid* or *interstitial fluid*, it carries nutrients, oxygen, proteins, and hormones into the cells.

As the tissue fluid leaves the cells, it takes some waste products with it, including protein molecules that were created within the cells. These protein molecules are important to the body and must be returned to the cardio-vascular system. Because they are too large to pass through the wall of the blood capillaries, these molecules are transported by the lymphatic system.

Ninety percent of the tissue fluid reenters the blood capillaries and continues its journey as plasma. The remaining ten percent of this fluid is now known as *lymph*. Lymph acts as a garbage collector and picks up debris including dead blood cells, pathogens, toxins, cancer cells, and the protein molecules that were left behind by the departing tissue fluid.[2] It is because of the presence of these protein molecules that lymph is described as being a *protein-rich fluid*. Lymph does not contain red blood cells or platelets. Lymph does contain clotting factors and will clot, although not as readily as blood.

How Lymph Becomes Protein-Rich

Proteins in food are broken down by the digestive tract. These components enter the bloodstream and are transported throughout the body by the blood plasma. *Plasma* is the liquid portion of blood.

Proteins and other nutrients leave the blood capillaries with the plasma that becomes tissue fluid. The tissue fluid carries nutrients into the cells. The cells use these components to create larger protein molecules.

Some of the larger proteins that leave the cells with the waste tissue fluid are too large to reenter the blood capillaries. The lymphatic system collects these waste proteins and processes them through the lymph nodes before they are recycled into the cardiovascular system.

The lymphatic fluid that accumulates in lymphedema is referred to as being protein-rich because it contains these unprocessed proteins.

Lymph Circulation

Lymph makes a one-way journey from the interstitial spaces to the lymphatic ducts located at the terminus. The *terminus* is the triangular-shaped indentation on each side at the base of the neck. It is formed in front by the clavicle (collarbone), on the side by the neck, and in the back by the top of the shoulder muscle, see Figure IV-7 on page 233.

As the lymph is transported upward, it passes through lymph nodes where it is filtered and processed to remove impurities. In the terminus the lymphatic ducts empty into the subclavian veins, which are located just under the collarbones. When lymph returns to the venous circulation, it once again becomes blood plasma.

How Fat Affects the Flow of Lymph *

As weight is gained, existing fat cells expand and more fat cells are added. Despite this increase in the number of cells, the body does not form additional lymph vessels. Factors placing additional stress on the lymphatic system include:

☐ Increasing the quantity of waste to be removed.

☐ Obstructing and slowing the flow of lymph through the fat layers, causing lymph to pool in the tissues.

☐ Trapping stagnant waste products in the tissues longer which increases the risk of infection and fibrosis.

☐ Causing lymph to travel further before it can return to the cardiovascular system.

☐ Pressing on lymph nodes and interfering with their function. For example, a large overlapping belly puts pressure on the lymph nodes in the groin.

*Note: our understanding of how fat functions is changing rapidly. This description is based on information available in early 2005.

Lymphatic structures that are located near, or just under, the skin are referred to as *superficial lymphatics.* Those structures located further within the body are referred to as *deep lymphatics.*

Lymphatic Capillaries

Lymph leaves the interstitial spaces by entering the *lymphatic capillaries,* which are also known as *initial lymphatics* or *absorbing lymphatic vessels.* Millions of these tiny capillaries are grouped together in mesh-like formations throughout the body.

Approximately 70 percent of the lymphatic capillaries are superficial. *Superficial* means located near, or just under, the skin. The remaining 30 percent, known as *deep lymphatic capillaries,* surround most of the body's organs.[3]

A lymphatic capillary begins as a blind-ended tube with walls that are only one cell in thickness. Each of these cells is fastened to the nearby tissue by an *anchoring filament.* As the tissues move, the filament forces the cells apart and allows lymph to enter the lymphatic capillary.[4]

Lymphatic Pre-Collectors and Collectors

The lymph flows from the lymphatic capillary into a *pre-collector,* which has walls that are about three cells thick. The pre-collectors merge into thicker vessels known as *collectors* and these eventually merge to form large vessels known as lymphatic trunks or ducts.

Lymphatic Trunks

The *lymphatic trunks,* the largest lymphatic vessels, are located deeper within the body near blood vessels. These vessels contain valves that are similar in structure to those found in veins. The purpose of these valves is to permit lymph to only flow upward (see Figure IV-5 on page 231).

The segment of the vessel between two valves is called an *angion* or *lymphangion.* The smooth muscles in the walls contract in a wave-like motion at a rate of one contraction every eight to twelve seconds. This rate of motion, which equals five-to-seven contractions per minute, pushes the lymph forward and helps to draw more lymph into the capillaries.[5]

As the lymph flows upward through the body it receives more help from the action of deep breathing, the motion of nearby blood vessels, and the movements of active muscles.

Lymph Nodes

Lymphatic vessels pass through lymph nodes where the lymph is filtered and processed before it returns to the cardiovascular system. There are 400 to 700 lymph nodes located throughout the body. About half of these nodes are located in the abdomen (see Figure IV-8 on page 234). Other nodes are clustered in the three major groups listed below, in groups located around major joints, or located singly along the lymphatic vessels. The three major groups of lymph nodes are (see also Figure IV-3):

- **Cervical lymph nodes** along the sides of the neck (see Figure IV-7). *Cervical* means relating to the neck.

- **Axillary lymph nodes** in the armpits (see Figure IV-6). *Axillary* means relating to the armpits.

- **Inguinal lymph nodes** located in the groin (see Figure IV-10). *Inguinal* means relating to the groin.

Structures and Functions of the Lymph Nodes

Lymph nodes are bean-shaped structures (see Figure IV-4 on page 230) surrounded by a **protective capsule**.[6] Lymph nodes range in size from as small as a pinhead to as large as an olive. Lymph nodes may become enlarged when they are fighting an infection.

The primary function of the lymph nodes is to act as defensive barriers against infections and malignant disorders by filtering lymph and destroying pathogens.[7] *Lymphocytes*, specialized white blood cells that defend against non-self or altered cells, are concentrated in the lymph nodes and produce *antibodies* that circulate through the blood and bind to non-self substances.

Lymph nodes contain a mesh of tissue tightly packed with lymphocytes and macrophages. As lymph is filtered through this mesh, harmful microorganisms are attacked and destroyed.

Each part of the node has a specific role:

- Lymph carrying waste flows into the node through **afferent lymphatic vessels** around the outer surface. *Afferent* means toward.

- The lymph flows through the **cortex** of the node where lymphocytes engulf and destroy damaged cells, cancer cells, and foreign particles such as bacteria and viruses. The *cortex* is the outer portion. Lymphocytes block or slow the spread of cancer until the node is overwhelmed by the disease.

- Next, the lymph flows into the **medulla** of the node. The *medulla* is the central portion. Here the lymph is filtered to remove waste products and about 40 percent of its liquid content is removed.

- The filtered lymph leaves through **efferent vessels** that connect to other lymph nodes and the lymphatic trunks. *Efferent* means away from.

The Transport of Lymph from the Legs

The upward flow of lymph from the feet to the trunk depends largely on the motion of nearby muscles and joints during exercise and other activities. This motion stimulates both the superficial and deep lymph flow (see Figures IV-10 and IV-11).

Muscle Pumps

The muscles that are most helpful in stimulating this upward flow are known as *major muscle pumps*. The major muscle pumps of the legs are the plantar muscles on the bottoms of the feet, the calf muscles in the lower leg, and the thigh muscles in the upper leg.[8] *Plantar* means relating to the sole of the foot.

Joint Pumps

The bending and straightening of the larger joints also stimulate the upward flow of lymph and these joints are known as *major joint pumps*. The major joint pumps in the lower body are the ankles, knees, and hips.[9]

The Transport of Lymph Through the Trunk

Major lymphatic vessels carry lymph upward from each leg into the trunk. Here these vessels merge to form the cisterna chyli (see Figure IV-9). The *cisterna chyli* is a small pouch located below the diaphragm that temporarily stores lymph as it travels upward from the legs and lower trunk.

From the cisterna chyli, the *thoracic duct* carries lymph upward through the chest. The thoracic duct transports lymph from both legs, the lower portion of the trunk, the left quadrant of the chest, plus the left side of the head and neck.

The thoracic duct carries lymph to the terminus at the base of the left side of the neck. Here it empties into the left subclavian vein and the lymph returns to the venous circulation as plasma.

Unequal Drainage Areas

A unique feature of the lymphatic system is that it is divided into very unequal drainage areas as shown in Figure IV-3. The upper right quadrant drains on the right side and the other three quadrants, including both lower extremities, drains on the left side.

The *right lymphatic duct* is much smaller than the left duct and removes lymph from the right hand and arm, upper right quadrant of the trunk, and the right half of the head and neck to the terminus on the right side of the neck. At the terminus, it connects into the right subclavian vein and returns the lymph to the venous circulation as plasma (see Figure IV-6).

Figure IV-3: Quadrants and groups of lymph nodes

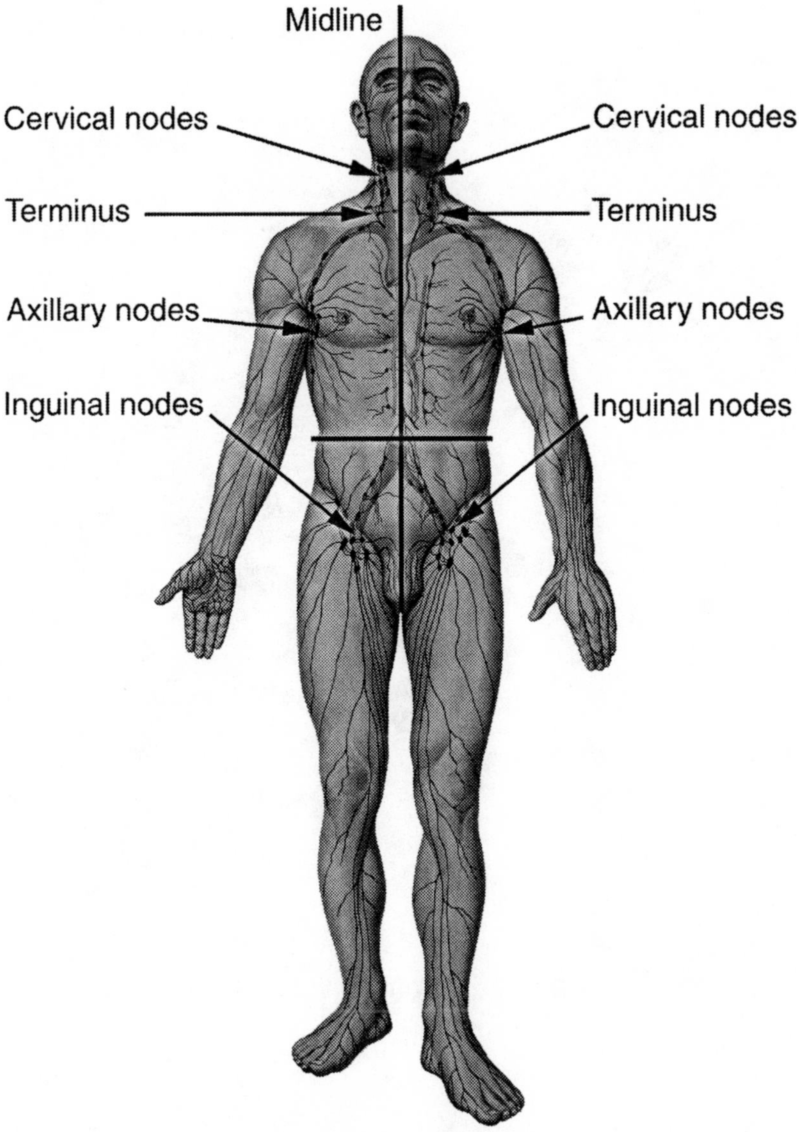

Midline

Cervical nodes

Cervical nodes

Terminus

Terminus

Axillary nodes

Axillary nodes

Inguinal nodes

Inguinal nodes

Figure IV-4: Structures of a lymph node.

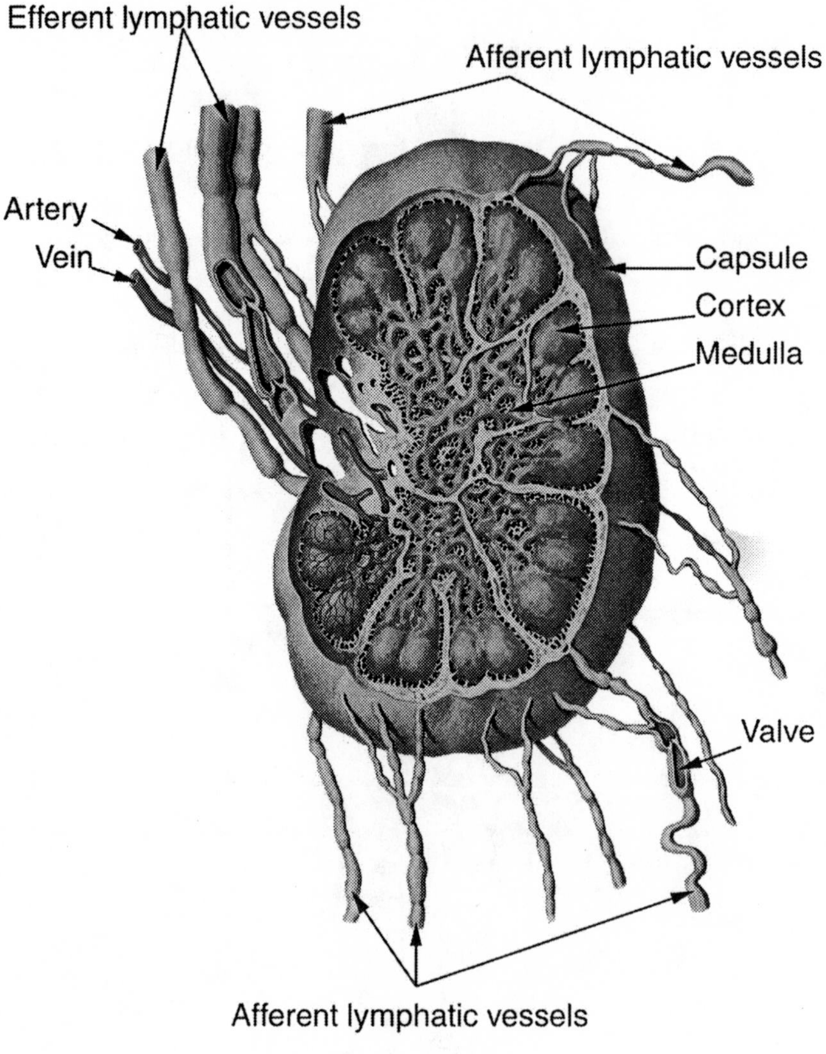

Efferent lymphatic vessels

Afferent lymphatic vessels

Artery

Vein

Capsule

Cortex

Medulla

Valve

Afferent lymphatic vessels

Figure IV-5: Structures of a vein and lymphatic vessel compared.

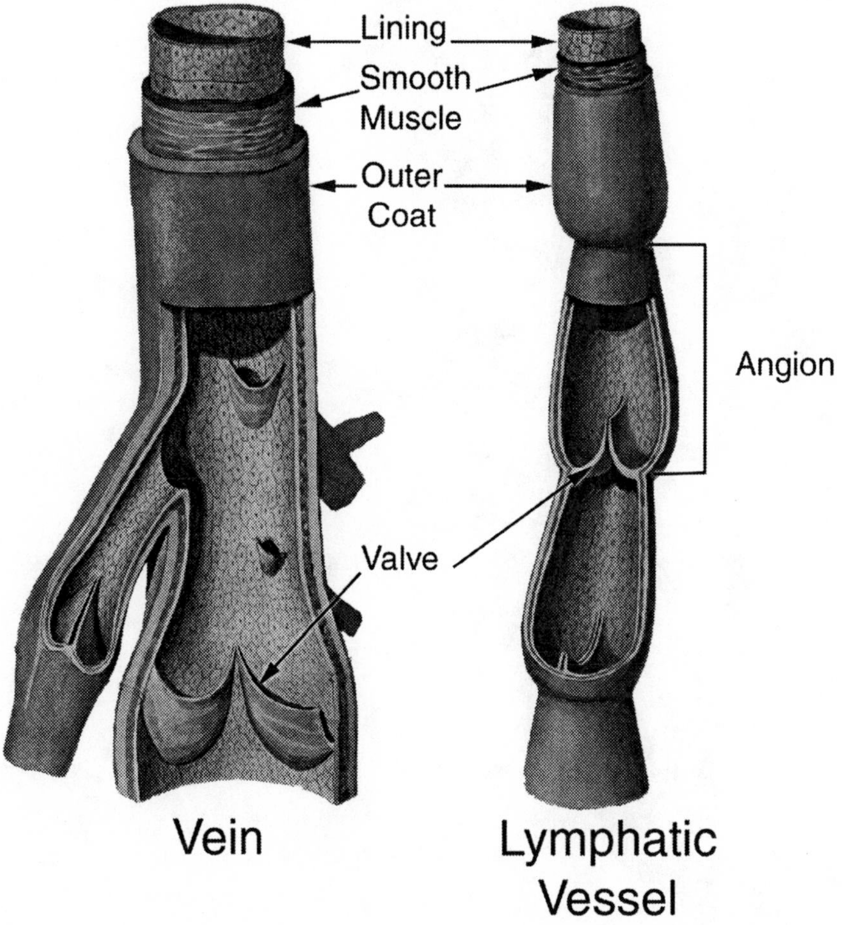

Lining

Smooth Muscle

Outer Coat

Angion

Valve

Vein

Lymphatic Vessel

Figure IV-6: Deep lymphatic structures of the arm.

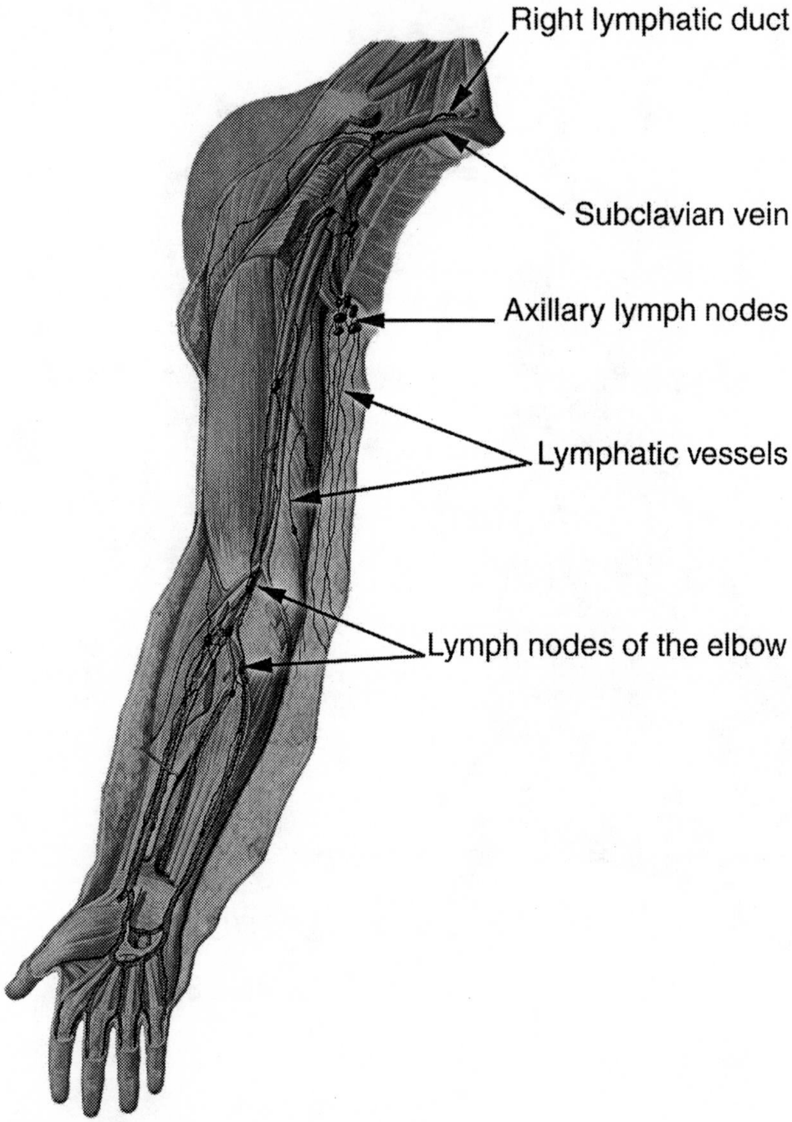

Right lymphatic duct

Subclavian vein

Axillary lymph nodes

Lymphatic vessels

Lymph nodes of the elbow

Figure IV-7: Lymphatic structures of the neck and upper body.

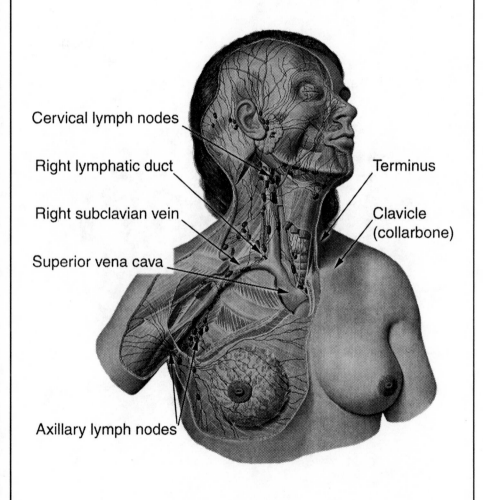

Cervical lymph nodes

Right lymphatic duct

Right subclavian vein

Superior vena cava

Terminus

Clavicle (collarbone)

Axillary lymph nodes

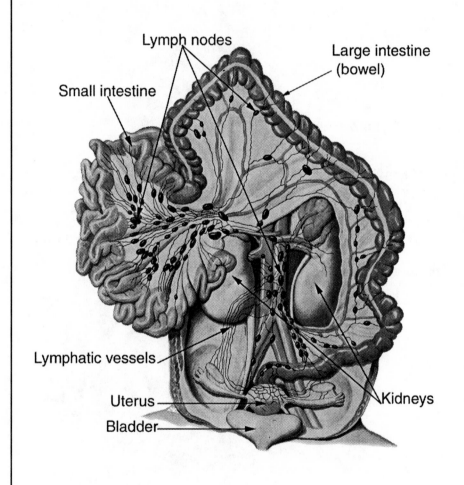

Figure IV-8: Major structures of the lower abdomen.

Lymph nodes

Large intestine (bowel)

Small intestine

Lymphatic vessels

Uterus

Bladder

Kidneys

Figure IV-9: Deep lymphatic structures of the trunk (frontal view).

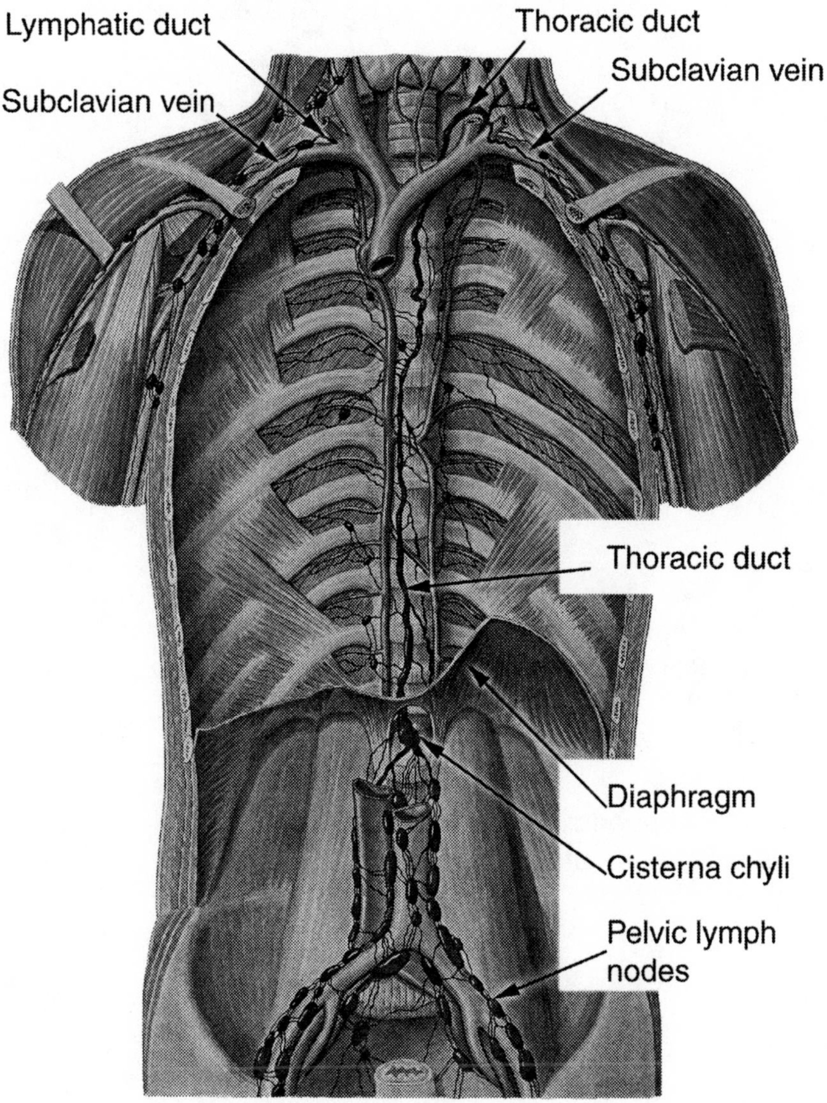

Lymphatic duct

Subclavian vein

Thoracic duct

Subclavian vein

Thoracic duct

Diaphragm

Cisterna chyli

Pelvic lymph nodes

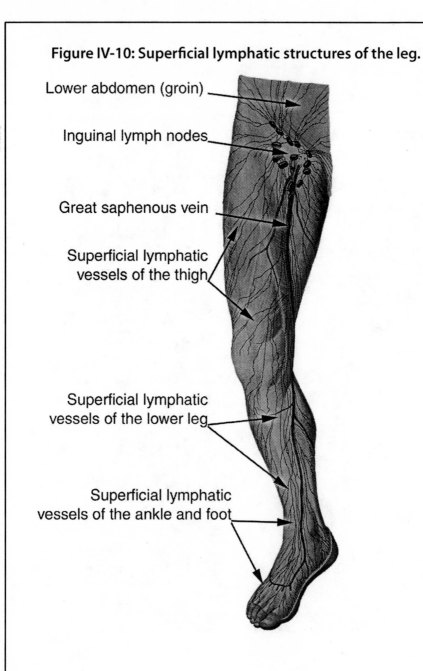

Figure IV-10: Superficial lymphatic structures of the leg.

Lower abdomen (groin)

Inguinal lymph nodes

Great saphenous vein

Superficial lymphatic vessels of the thigh

Superficial lymphatic vessels of the lower leg

Superficial lymphatic vessels of the ankle and foot

Figure IV-11: Muscle and joint pumps of the leg, rear view.

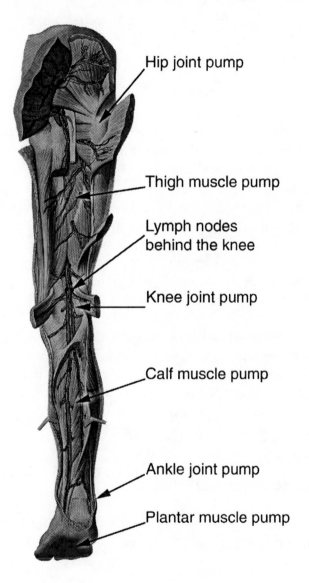

Hip joint pump

Thigh muscle pump

Lymph nodes
behind the knee

Knee joint pump

Calf muscle pump

Ankle joint pump

Plantar muscle pump

How Lymphedema Treatment Works

Lymphedema treatment works by manipulating the lymphatic capillaries and ducts to stimulate the flow of lymph through the body. Light pressure and slow movements mimic the natural movements of the lymphatic vessels.

Manual Lymph Drainage typically follows the normal direction and path of flow within the lymphatic system. Lymph drainage starts at the terminus, which is the place where the large lymphatic ducts empty into the subclavian veins at the base of the neck.

Lymph drainage works from the terminus down the trunk and out to the extremities, and then back to the terminus in the reverse sequence. By starting at the terminus, MLD creates space within the lymphatic vessels for the fluid that will be drained from other parts of the body. If congestion develops during MLD, the therapist may drain the terminus and major groups of nodes repeatedly.

In situations where a path is obstructed, a therapist may massage across the midline and direct the flow of lymph from the affected quadrant to the intact quadrant. For example, if the axillary nodes in the right armpit have been damaged, the therapist may massage the back and stroke across the spine, going from the right side to the left side, so that lymph can drain via the intact axillary nodes on the left side.

Lymphatic System Dysfunctions

Each cause of lymphedema interferes with the function of the lymphatic system in a different way. Lymphedema may result from a combination of these causes:

*   **Primary lymphedema** is an inherited condition with several variations (see Chapter 1). A wide variety of lymphatic developmental abnormalities have been observed including the congential absence of lymphatic vessels, or more commonly, *hypoplasia* where there are fewer lymphatics present and they are smaller than normal.[10]

- **Tissue injuries** destroy lymphatic vessels. As wounds heal, lymphatic capillaries grow by sprouting from existing lymphatics. The ability to regenerate varies with the consistency of the connective tissue and the size of the injured area. Inflammation can destroy lymphatics and infection interferes with lymphatic regeneration, possibly due to fibrosis. Large scars and burns (including radiation) often lead to lymphatic impairment of the skin.

- **Lymph node dissection** is a surgical procedure in which lymph nodes are removed, **lymph node biopsy** is a procedure in which parts of a lymph node are removed either surgically or with a sampling device. Both procedures destroy lymph nodes and lymphatic vessels, disrupting the flow of lymph through the affected area. In cases of breast cancer the axillary nodes are damaged and lymphatic drainage from the arm is disrupted; for prostate and other pelvic cancers the inguinal nodes are damaged impairing lymphatic drainage from the legs.

- **Obesity and lipedema** increase the amount of fat in the body. Lymphatic vessels in the skin drain through the layer of fat located just under the skin (subcutaneous fat). As this fat layer becomes thicker and denser it becomes harder for the lymph to pass through the fat. Subcutaneous fat separates the skin from the large muscles and may interfere with the natural pumping action of the muscles.

- **Inactivity, paralysis or muscle damage** decrease the pumping action of the large muscles and joints that normally stimulates the drainage of lymph.

- **Filariasis** is caused by parasitic worms (filariae) that live in the lymphatic vessels and cause lymphatic vessel dilation and blockage. Filariasis is a tropical disease spread by mosquitoes. Treatment includes medication to kill the parasites and prevent infections due to breaks in the skin, combined with other lymphedema treatments.

Stories of the Lymph Notes Team

We've learned a lot since starting Lymph Notes:

- People all over the world live with lymphedema. Thanks to the Internet, we've heard from many of them, and their families.

- Lymphedema may be obscure but it is not rare; approximately 5 million Americans and 170 million people worldwide are living with lymphedema.

- Lymphedema has many variations and secondary lymphedema has many causes.

- Therapy is the key to living well and lymphedema therapists do not receive either the respect or rewards that they deserve.

- Research is underway, government grants are available, and there is a new journal of Lymphatic Research and Biology; thanks in part to the efforts of the Lymphatic Research Foundation (www.lymphaticresearch.org).

- Dragon boat racers and other people with lymphedema are defying the conventional wisdom (see Chapter 16); hopefully this will lead to new understanding and lymphedema treatments.

We would like to hear from you (via LymphNotes.com), please:

- Share your stories and tips for living well with lymphedema.

- List your treatment center or support group in our directory.

Notes and References

Chapter 1—What is Lymphedema

[1] Dale, R. F. "The Inheritance of Primary Lymphedema." **Journal of Medical Genetics** 22:274-278, 1985.

[2] Chikly, B. **Silent Waves: Theory and Practice of Lymphatic Drainage Therapy.** I.H.H. Publishing, 2001, p. 170.

[3] Casley-Smith, J.R. and Casley-Smith, J.R. **Modern Treatment for Lymphoedema, 5-E.** The Lymphoedema Association of Australia, 1997, p. 95.

[4] Levinson, K.L., Feingold, E., et al *"Age of onset in hereditary lymphedema."* **J. Pediatr.** 2003 Jun;142 (6):704-8.

[5] Feldman, J.L. "Management of Childhood and Adolescent Lymphedema." **Lymph Link,** Vol 16:2 April-June 2004, p. 1.

[6] Stewart, P.J. "When It Isn't Lymphedema." **Lymph Link,** Vol 16, No 3, 2004, p. 1.

[7] Lasinski, B. "The Lymphatic System Pathology" in Goodman, C.C, Boissonnault, W.G., and Fuller K.S. **Pathology: Implications for the Physical Therapist 2-E.** Saunders, 2003, p. 485.

[8] Casley-Smith, J.R. and Casley-Smith, J.R. **Modern Treatment for Lymphoedema, 5-E.** The Lymphoedema Association of Australia, 1997, p. 94.

[9] Chikly, B. **Silent Waves: Theory and Practice of Lymphatic Drainage Therapy.** I.H.H. Publishing, 2001, p. 39-40.

[10] Wittlinger, G. and Wittlinger, H. **Textbook of Dr. Vodder's Manual Lymph Drainage, Volume 1: Basic Course.** Karl F. Haug Verlag, 1998, p. 77-78.

Chapter 2—The Diagnosis of Lymphedema

[1] Rockson, S.G. "Evaluation and Management of Lymphedema." **Am J. Med,** March 2001;110:288-95.

[2] Szuba, A, et al. "The Third Circulation: Radionuclide Lymphoscintigraphy in the Evaluation of Lymphedema."*JNM*, 44:1, January 2003.

[3] Lasinski, B. "The Lymphatic System Pathology" in Goodman, C.C, Boissonnault, W.G., and Fuller K.S. **Pathology Implications for the Physical Therapist 2-E.** Saunders, 2003 p. 484-485.

Chapter 3—How Lymphedema is Treated

[1] Kelly, D. G. **A Primer on Lymphedema.** Prentice Hall, 2002, p. 68.

[2] Kelly, D. G. **A Primer on Lymphedema.** Prentice Hall, 2002, p. 69.

[3] Chikly, B. **Silent Waves: Theory and Practice of Lymphatic Drainage Therapy.** I.H.H. Publishing, 2001, p. 111.

[4] "The Diagnosis and Treatment of Peripheral Lymphedema: Consensus Document of the International Society of Lymphology." **Lymphology** 36, 2003, p. 84-91.

[5] Muscari-Lin, E. "Truncal Lymphedema." **Lymphlink**. Jan-Mar 2004, 16(1).

[6] The Kinesio Taping® Association (www.kinesiotaping.com).

Chapter 4—Finding Quality Lymphedema Treatment

[1] "Position Paper on the Training of Lymphedema Therapists." National Lymphedema Network. Nov. 2003.

[2] Brown, H.S. "Developing a Suitable and Functional Lymphedema Management Program." **Lymph Link,** Vol 16, No 3, 2004 p. 7-25.

Chapter 5—Insurance and Reimbursement Issues

[1] COBRA (www.dol.gov/dol/topic/health-plans/cobra.htm/)

[2] HIPAA (www.cms.hhs.gov/hipaa)

[3] ADA (www. ada/gov)

[4] FMLA (www.dol.gov/esa/whd/fmla/)

[5] WHCRA (www.dol.gov/ebsa/publications/whcra.html)

Chapter 6—Complications of Lymphedema

[1] Lehrer, M. "Cellulitis." **MedlinePlus Medical Encyclopedia,** National Library of Medicine, 2002.

[2] Landro, L. "Healthy People Are at Growing Risk from Staph Infections." **The Wall Street Journal,** October 9, 2003, p. D1–D3.

[3] Kotton, C. "Erysipelas." **MedlinePlus Medical Encyclopedia,** National Library of Medicine, 2002.

[4] "Nail Fungus." **Lymph Links**, Vol 13:3, 2001.

[5] MacLaren, J.A. "Skin changes in lymphoedema: pathophysiology and management options." **Int J Palliat Nurs.** 2001 Aug;7(8):381-8.

[6] Chikly, B. Silent Waves: Theory and Practice of Lymphatic Drainage Therapy. I.H.H. Publishing, 2001, p. 208.

[7] Stubblefield, H. "Rotator cuff tendonitis in lymphedema: a retrospective case series." Arch Phys Med Rehabil. 2004 Dec;85(12):1939-42.

[8] Andrews, L.R., Cofield RH, O'Driscoll SW. "Shoulder arthroplasty in patients with prior mastectomy for breast cancer." J Shoulder Elbow Surg. 2000 Sep-Oct;9(5):386-8.

Chapter 7—Lymphedema and Other Conditions

[1] McCracken, N. "Considering Co-Morbidities in the Treatment of Lymphedema." **Lymph Link**, Vol 16, No 3, 2004, p. 5-7.

[2] Macdonald, J.M., et al. "Lymphedema, Lipedema, and the Open Wound: the role of compression therapy." **Surg Clin North Am.** 2003 Jun;83(3):639-58.

[3] Gold, R. "Das Lipödem-Krankheit oder Fehlanlage?" **Zeitschrift für Lymphology** 1996; 20:73-75. Schattaurt GmbH.

[4] Grossman, S. "Congestive Heart Failure and Pulmonary Edema." E. Medicine January 2002. (www.emedicine.com/EMERG/topic108.htm).

[5] Lindholm, C. Bergsten, A, Berglund E. "Lymphedema and Diabetes." **J Wound Care** 1999 Jan:8 (1):5-10.

[6] Brennan, M J., Weitz, J. "Lymphedema 30 years after Radical Mastectomy." **Am J. Physical Rehabil** 1992:71:12-14.

Chapter 8—The Emotional Challenges of Lymphedema

[1] Velanovick, V., Szymanski, W. "Quality of Life of Breast Cancer Patients with Lymphedema." **Amer Journal of Surgery**, 1999; 177(3): 184-187.

[2] Abercrombie, B. **Writing Out the Storm: Reading and Writing Your Way Through Serious Illness or Injury.** St. Martin's Griffin, 2002.

[3] Pennebaker, J. **Opening Up: The Healing Power of Expressing Emotions.** The Guilford Press, 1997.

[4] Stone, D., Patton, B., Heen, S. **Difficult Conversations: How to Discuss What Matters Most.** Delacorte Press, 1996.

Section II—Additional References

Centers for Disease Control and Prevention MRSA Fact Sheet June 2004. (www.cdc.gov/ncidod/hip/Aresist/mrsafaq.htm)

"Lipedema Complicated by Lymphedema of the Abdominal Wall and Lower Limbs" by A. Zelikovski, M. Haddad, et al. **Lymphology** 33 (2000) 43-46

"Lymphedema" by D. R Revis, Jr. MD. www.emedicine.com. Updated September 6, 2002.

"Lymphedema and Quality of Life in Survivors of Life in Survivors of Early-Stage Breast Cancer" by S.M.Beaulac, L.A. McNair, et al. **Arch Surg.** 2002:1371253-1257.

"Lymphedema Management" by A.L Cheville, et al. **Semin Radiat Oncol.** 2003 Jul:13(3):290-301.

"Lymphedema Strategies for Management" by S.R. Cohen, D.K. Payne, and R.S. Tunkel. Cancer Rehabilitation in the New Millennium, Supplement to **Cancer.**

"Management of Childhood and Adolescent Lymphedema" by J.F. Feldman. **Lymph Link** Vol 16:2, April-June 2004. p. 1-26.

"The Diagnosis and Treatment of Peripheral Lymphedema: Consensus Document of the International Society of Lymphology." **Lymphology** 36 (2003) p. 84-91.

"When It Isn't Lymphedema" by P.J.B. Stewart. **Lymph Link**, Vol 16, No 3 2004 p 1-2.

A Primer on Lymphedema by D. G. Kelly. Prentice Hall, 2002.

Centers for Disease Control and Prevention (www.cdc.gov).

Coping with Lymphedema by J. Swirsky and D. S. Nannery. Avery Publishing Group, 1998.

Diseases of the Lymphatics by N. Browse, K.G. Burnand, and P. Mortimer. Arnold Publishers, 2003.

Living Beyond Breast Cancer: A Survivor's Guide for When Treatment Ends and the Rest of Your Life Begins by M.C. Weiss and E. Weiss. Times Books, 1998, p. 134-143.

Lymphedema Diagnosis and Therapy by H. Weissleder and C. Suchard (eds.). Viavital Verlag GmbH, 2001.

Chapter 9—Skin, Nail, and Foot Care

[1] **First Aid Guide - Mayo Clinic.com** available at www.mayoclinic.com

Chapter 10—Self-Massage

[1] Burt, J. and White, G. **Lymphedema: A Breast Cancer Patient's Guide to Prevention and Healing**. Hunter House Publishers, 1999, p. 55-62.

[2] Kasseroller, R. **Compendium of Dr. Vodder's Manual Lymph Drainage.** Haug Verlag, 1998, p 50.

[3] de Godoy, J.M Torres, C.A. and Godoy, M.F. "Self-drainage lymphatic technique" **Angiology.** 2001 Aug:52(8):573-4.

[4] Burt, J. and White, G. **Lymphedema: A Breast Cancer Patient's Guide to Prevention and Healing.** Hunter House Publishers, 1999, p. 66-68.

Chapter 11—Self-Bandaging

[1] Klose, G. **Lymphedema Bandaging.** Lohmann Rauscher, p. 14.

[2] Földi, E. and Földi, M. **Lymphedema Management Today.** BSN-Jobst, p. 26.

Chapter 12—Home Exercise Program

[1] Whitfield, P. **The Human Body Explained.** Henry Holt and Company, 1995, p. 128.

[2] Lasinski, B. "The Lymphatic System" in Goodman, C.C., Boissonnault, W.G., and Fuller, K.S. **Pathology: Implications for the Physical Therapist 2-E.** Saunders, 2003, p. 498-499.

[3] **MediFocus Guide: Lymphedema.** Medifocus.com, Inc., 2004, p. 13.

[4] Chikly, B. **Silent Waves: Theory and Practice of Lymph Drainage Theory.** I.H.H. Publishing 2001 p. 283.

Chapter 13—Aquatic Exercises

[1] Harris, S. "Getting (and Staying) Aerobically Fit through Swimming!" **Active Living** Vol 3:#3, June 2002.

[2] White, M. **Water Exercises.** Human Kinetics, 1995.

[3] Rymal, C. "Can patients at risk for lymphedema use hot tubs?" **Clin J Oncol Nurs.** 2002 Nov-Dec;6(6):369.

Chapter 14—Nutrition Tips

No notes

Chapter 15—Keeping a Health Journal

No notes

Chapter 16—Having Fun

[1] Harris, S.R. and Niesen-Vertommen, S.L. "Challenging the myth of exercise-induced lymphedema: A series of case reports." **Journal of Surgical Oncology** April 2000.

[2] Unruk A.M, and Elvin, N. "In the eye of the dragon: Women's experience of breast cancer and the occupation of dragon boat racing." **Canadian Association Occupational Therapists Abstracts.** Vol 71, No 3, June 2004.

[3] NLN Air Travel Position Paper, May 2004.

[4] Tavakoli, S.A. and Yates, W.R. "Sauna and hot tub warnings." **Psychosomatics.** May-Jun;44(3):261-2, 2003.

[5] Chikley, B. **Silent Waves Theory and Practice of Lymph Drainage Therapy.** I.H.H. Publishing, 2001, p. 281.

[6] Lebed-Davis, S. **Thriving after Breast Cancer: Essential Healing Exercises for Body and Mind.** Broadway Books, 2002.

Section III—Additional References

Compendium of Dr. Vodder's Manual Lymph Drainage by R. Kasseroller. Karl F. Haug Verlag, 1998.

Compression Step by Step: Practical Bandaging Instructions by P. Staudinger. Beiersdorf Medical Bibliotek, 1991.

First Aid for Burn Care by D. Willoughby. PageWise, 2002.

Lymphedema Bandaging. Lohmann Rauscher pamphlet.

Lymphedema Self-Care Manual by P. Tubbs-Gingerich. Moon Lith Press, 2003.

Oedeem en Oedeemtherapie by H.P.M. Verdonk et al. Bohn, Stafleu, Van Loghum. Houten/Diegem, 2000.

Section IV—Understanding the Lymphatic System

[1] Casley-Smith, J.R. and Casley-Smith, J.R. **Modern Treatment for Lymphoedema,** 5-E. The Lymphoedema Association of Australia, Inc., 1997, p. 14.

[2] Lasinski, B. "The Lymphatic System in Pathology." in Goodman CC, et al. **Pathology Implications for the Physical Therapist** 2-E. Saunders, 2003, p 477.

[3] Casley-Smith, J.R. and Casley-Smith, J.R. **Modern Treatment for Lymphoedema,** 5-E. The Lymphoedema Association of Australia, Inc., 1997, p. 25.

[4] Cohen, S.R., Payne, D.K. et al. "Lymphedema Strategies for Management." **Cancer Rehabilitation in the New Millennium,** Supplement to Cancer 2001, 980-987.

[5] Kasseroller, R. **Compendium of Dr. Vodder's Manual Lymph Drainage.** Haug, 1998.

[6] Casley-Smith, J.R. and Casley-Smith, J.R. **Modern Treatment for Lymphoedema, 5-E.** The Lymphoedema Association of Australia, Inc., 1997, p. 20.

[7] Lasinski, B. "The Lymphatic System in Pathology." in Goodman CC, et al. **Pathology Implications for the Physical Therapist 2-E.** Saunders, 2003, p.484.

[8] Földi, M., Földi, E. and Kubik, S. eds. **Textbook of Lymphology for Physicians and Lymphedema Therapists.** Urban & Fischer, 2003, p 514-516.

[9] Földi, M., Földi, E. and Kubik, S. eds. **Textbook of Lymphology for Physicians and Lymphedema Therapists.** Urban & Fischer, 2003, p. 514.

[10] Kelly, D. G. **A Primer on Lymphedema.** Prentice Hall, 2002, p. 30.

Section IV—Additional References

Atlas of Human Anatomy. TAJ Books Ltd, 2002.

Atlas of the Human Body by T. Takahashi. Harper Collins, 1994.

Basic Lymphoedema Management: Treatment and Prevent of Problems Associated with Lymphatic Filariasis by Dreyer, et al. Hollis Publishing Company. 2002.

Body Structures and Functions 9-Ed by A. Scott and E. Fong. Delmar Learning, 1998, p. 240-241.

"Current Concepts in Lymphedema Management" by Mary Sieggreen and Ronald Kline. **Advances in Skin & Wound Care.** Vol 17 No 4 May 2004.

Delmar's Fundamentals of Anatomy and Physiology by D. Rizzo. Delmar Learning, 2001.

Human Physiology and Mechanisms of Disease 6-Ed by A.C. Guyton and J.E. Hall. W.B Saunders Company, 1997.

"Lymphatics at the crossroads of angiogenesis and lymphangiogenesis" by Claudio Scavelli et. al. **J. Anat.** (2004) 204 pp433-449.

Lymphedema (PDQ) Health Professional Version. National Cancer Institute. Last modified 08/19/2004 available at www.cancer.gov

"Pathophysiology of secondary lymphedema" by M. J. W. Hismann and U. K. Franzeck. **Phlebolymphology** 23 available at www.servier.com.

"Postsurgical lymphedema - why does it occur?" by P. S. Mortimer. **Phlebolymphology** 32 available at www.servier.com.

Structure and Function in Man, 5-Ed by S. Jacob and C. Francone. W.B. Saunders Company, 1982, p 430-435.

Structure and Function of the Human Body 11th Ed by G. Thibodeaua and K. Patton. Mosby, 2000, p. 308-312.

Textbook of Dr. Vodder's Manual Lymph Drainage, Volume 1: Basic Course by G. Wittlinger and H. Wittlinger. Karl F. Haug Verlag, 1998, p. 46-53.

The Human Body Explained by P. Whitfield ed. Henry Holt and Company, 1995.

Index

About the Authors

Ann Ehrlich is a professional medical writer who also has secondary lymphedema following breast cancer treatment. Ann brings to this book her personal "need to know" on living well with lymphedema.

Alma Vinjé-Harrewijn, PT, CLT is a licensed physical therapist with more than 15 years of experience and postgraduate training in manual lymph drainage using the techniques of Vodder, Földi, Chikly, and others. Alma brings to this book many practical techniques, especially for self care, based on her years of experience helping people live well with lymphedema. She is a member of the International Society of Lymphology and the NVFL (the Dutch association for physical therapy specialists in lymphology) and writes a regular column for **Oedeminus**, the NVFL journal.

Elizabeth McMahon, PhD is a clinical psychologist who brings to this book over 25 years of experience helping patients, many of whom have chronic medical conditions. She shares her expertise in helping these individuals learn new skills for managing anxiety, depression, and other emotional issues that can be part of living well with a chronic condition like lymphedema.

Do you have a lymphedema support group?

No To find a support group, check the Lymphedema
Resources directory on LymphNotes.com
and/or
Join our online support group in the Lymph Notes
Forums: LymphNotes.com/bb/

Yes Be sure that your group is listed on Lymph Notes.
To add your group, e-mail the information to
groups@lymphnotes.com

Got Lymphedema? At risk for Lymphedema?

Get your free Lymphedema Wallet Card from
LymphNotes.com. Carry this card with your
insurance and ID cards to let emergency personnel
know about your condition.

To receive your free wallet card, please e-mail
cards@lymphnotes.com. Be sure to include your
postal address with your request.

Does your organization offer lymphedema treatment, garments, or products? Is your organization a Lymph Notes sponsor or listed in the Lymph Notes Directory?

Yes Thank you for your cooperation and support.

No You are missing a great opportunity to get your message in front of potential customers at the time when they are making purchase decisions. Contact sales@lymphnotes.com for information on sponsorship, or a free directory listing, now.

Are you a therapist or medical professional?

Register for Lymph Notes Professional Status and get:

- Listing as a Lymphedema Professional for yourself, and a link to your employer (if they are a sponsor).

- Access to the Medical Professionals Only forums.

- Pro status and a pro icon on your Forum posts.

Join Lymph Notes as a member, and then go to My Lymph Notes for details.

Printed in the United States
146714LV00003B/14/A

9 780976 480617